Outdoors
with **Kids**

- -

Maine, New Hampshire, and Vermont

75 OF THE BEST FAMILY HIKING, CAMPING, AND PADDLING TRIPS

ETHAN HIPPLE AND YEMAYA ST.CLAIR

Appalachian Mountain Club Books
Boston, Massachusetts

AMC is a nonprofit organization, and sales of AMC Books fund our mission of protecting the Northeast outdoors. If you appreciate our efforts and would like to become a member or make a donation to AMC, visit outdoors.org, call 800-372-1758, or contact us at Appalachian Mountain Club, 5 Joy Street, Boston, MA 02108.

outdoors.org/publications/books

Distributed by National Book Network.

Front cover photograph © Jerry and Marcy Monkman, EcoPhotography.com
Interior photographs by Ethan Hipple or Yemaya St.Clair © Appalachian Mountain Club, unless otherwise noted.
Maps by Ken Dumas © Appalachian Mountain Club
Cover design by Matt Simmons
Interior design by Joyce Weston

Library of Congress Cataloging-in-Publication Data

Hipple, Ethan.
  Outdoors with kids Maine, New Hampshire, and Vermont : 75 of the best family hiking, camping, and paddling trips / Ethan Hipple, Yemaya St. Clair.
    pages cm
  Summary: "This regional guide features 75 destinations in Northern New England where families can get outside, be active, and enjoy nature; includes tips for successful outings, informational maps, photos, and essays ranging from ecology to games on the go"-- Provided by publisher.
  ISBN 978-1-62842-003-6 (paperback) -- ISBN 1-62842-003-0 (paperback) 1. Outdoor recreation--New England--Guidebooks. 2. Family recreation--New England--Guidebooks. 3. Children--Travel--New England--Guidebooks. 4. New England--Guidebooks. I. St. Clair, Yemaya. II. Title.
  GV191.42.N3H57 2014
  796.50974--dc23
                    2014016987

The paper used in this publication meets the minimum requirements of the American National Standard for Information Sciences-Permanence of Paper for Printed Library Materials, ANSI Z39.48-1984. ∞

Outdoor recreation activities by their very nature are potentially hazardous. This book is not a substitute for good personal judgment and training in outdoor skills. Due to changes in conditions, use of the information in this book is at the sole risk of the user. The authors and the Appalachian Mountain Club assume no liability for accidents happening to, or injuries sustained by, readers who engage in the activities described in this book.

Interior pages contain 30% post-consumer recycled fiber.
Cover contains 10% post-consumer recycled fiber.
Printed in the United States of America,
using vegetable-based inks.

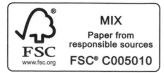

REGIONAL MAP

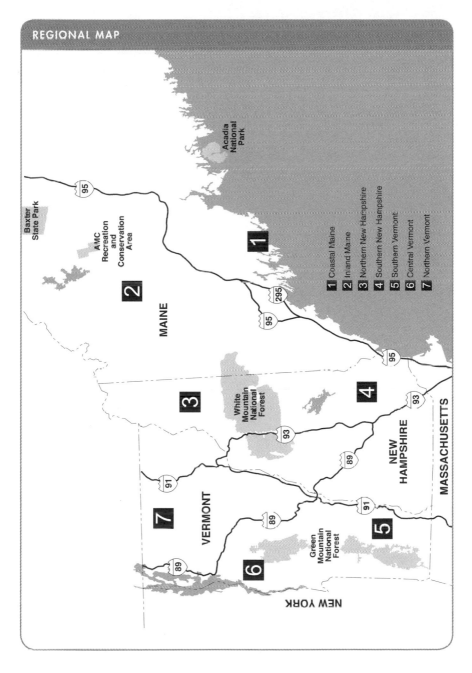

1 Coastal Maine
2 Inland Maine
3 Northern New Hampshire
4 Southern New Hampshire
5 Southern Vermont
6 Central Vermont
7 Northern Vermont

Acadia National Park

Baxter State Park

AMC Recreation and Conservation Area

MAINE

White Mountain National Forest

NEW HAMPSHIRE

MASSACHUSETTS

VERMONT

Green Mountain National Forest

NEW YORK

95 · 295 · 93 · 89 · 91

CONTENTS

SECTION 7: NORTHERN VERMONT

ESSAYS AND ACTIVITIES

AT-A-GLANCE TRIP PLANNER

# Trip	Page	Age	Difficulty*	Fee	Dog Friendly	Stroller Friendly
COASTAL MAINE						
1. Scarborough Marsh Audubon Center	2	5+	E–M		🐕	
2. Eastern Trail	4	All	E–M		🐕	🚼
3. Back Cove and Eastern Promenade Trails	7	All	E–M		🐕	🚼
4. Fore River Sanctuary and Jewell Falls	10	All	E		🐕	
5. Peaks Island	13	All	E		🐕	🚼
6. Mackworth Island	17	All	E	$	🐕	🚼
7. Gilsland Farm Audubon Center	20	All	E			
8. Bradbury Mountain	23	All	E–M	$	🐕	
9. Wolfe's Neck Woods State Park	25	All	E	$	🐕	🚼
10. Hermit Island	28	All	E–M	$		
11. Morse Mountain	31	All	E–M			🚼
12. Mount Battie	33	5+	M	$	🐕	
13. Penobscot Mountain	36	8+	C	$	🐕	
14. The Bubbles	39	All	E–M	$	🐕	
15. Carriage Roads	43	All	E–M	$	🐕	
16. Little Moose Island	46	All	E–M	$	🐕	
INLAND MAINE						
17. Douglas Mountain	50	5+	M	$		
18. Burnt Meadow Mountain	53	5+	M–C		🐕	
19. Pleasant Mountain	56	5+	M		🐕	
20. The Roost	58	All	E–M	$	🐕	
21. Table Rock	60	5+	M	$	🐕	
22. Borestone Mountain Audubon Sactuary	66	8+	M–C	$		

* E = Easy, M=Moderate, C=Challenging

Hike	Bike	Paddle/ Swim	Camp	Winter Trip	Highlights
🚶		🚣			Paddle Maine's largest saltwater marsh
🚶	🚴			🧢	Flat, off-road trail through woods and wetland
🚶	🚴			🧢	Off-road recreational trails through Portland
🚶	🚴		⛺	🧢	85 acres of trails and wildlife in Portland
🚶	🚴				Ride the ferry to a seaside bike path
🚶		🏊		🧢	Easy loop hike to tidal pools and a fairy village
🚶				🧢	Gentle trails and a nature center near Portland
🚶	🚴		⛺	🧢	Easy hiking to views; perfect introductory hike
🚶				🧢	Easy, accessible coastal and forested trails
🚶	🚴	🚣 🏊	⛺		Classic coastal Maine camping experience
🚶		🏊		🧢	Summit a mountain then head to the beach!
🚶					Hike to stone tower and coastal views
🚶					Varied, exciting terrain in Acadia National Park
🚶					Quick uphill hike to a glacial erratic and views
🚶	🚴				Broken-stone paths tour Acadia's landscape
🚶					Cross a land bridge for a quiet, wild island hike
🚶				🧢	Lookout to the Whites from a 1920s tower
🚶				🧢	Climb and scramble to stunning views
🚶				🧢	Summit southern Maine's tallest peak
🚶					Short trail in Evans Notch to views
🚶					Spectacular views along a Grafton Notch trail
🚶					Visit a nature center and scramble to a summit

Hike	Bike	Paddle/ Swim	Camp	Winter Trip	Highlights
✓		✓ (paddle/swim)		✓	Enjoy an AMC lodge and paddle a wild lake
✓		✓ (paddle/swim)	✓		Base camp and explore Baxter State Park
✓		✓ (paddle)	✓		Hike and paddle at this recreation resort
✓	✓	✓ (paddle/swim)		✓	Peaceful biking and paddling in Wolfeboro
✓		✓ (swim)			Open ridge hike to little-known peak
	✓	✓ (paddle/swim)			Mountain valley paddle, swimming, picnics
✓					Perfect hike for toddlers
		✓ (paddle/swim)			Easy river paddle with plenty of swimming
		✓ (swim)			Easy hike to incredible views of Squam Lake
✓		✓ (swim)	✓		Hike and camp; great views and waterfalls
✓					Could be the perfect New England loop hike
✓		✓ (swim)			A short hike to idyllic swimming holes
✓					Small-yet-mighty peak with a gentle grade
✓					Easy hiking to great views; great intro trip
		✓ (paddle/swim)			Idyllic paddling in the Kinsman Range
✓		✓ (swim)			Hike to waterfalls and a backcountry hut
✓	✓	✓ (swim)	✓	✓	Scenic biking in the White Mountains
		✓ (paddle/swim)	✓		Paddle and camp on a wild lake
✓			✓		Remote hike to mountaintop fire tower
✓			✓		Short hike to iconic granite dome
		✓ (paddle/swim)			Idyllic paddling with picnicking and fishing
✓		✓ (swim)			Magnificent views from a craggy peak
✓					Easy hike with great views
✓	✓	✓ (paddle/swim)	✓	✓	Gentle hiking to ponds and wetlands
		✓ (paddle/swim)			Wildlife viewing and paddling close to the city
✓	✓	✓ (swim)		✓	Scenic biking near Manchester
		✓ (paddle/swim)			Crystal clear waters and a hidden pond

Hike	Bike	Paddle/Swim	Camp	Winter Trip	Highlights
✓					Easy hike to panoramic views
✓					A very easy hike to spectacular views
✓			✓	✓	Excellent views and a mountaintop shelter
✓	✓	✓	✓		Bike then hike to waterfalls
✓	✓	✓ (paddle/swim)			Paddle, picnic, hike, and swim—all in one trip!
✓		✓	✓		A fun walk up a sunny ski area
✓		✓	✓	✓	Hike and camp in a serene farmland oasis
		✓ (paddle/swim)	✓		Connecticut River paddling to overnight camping on an island; access from VT and NH
✓					Pleasant hike from a charming village
✓		✓	✓		Unique waterfall and a peaceful lake
✓					High country in Vermont's rural farmlands
✓					Easy hike to west-facing ledges
✓					Stellar views from a 4,006-foot peak
✓	✓	✓	✓	✓	Bike through the heart of pastoral Vermont
✓					Easy hike to open ledges
✓		✓	✓		Mountain and pond loop hike
✓				✓	Easy hike to views of the Adirondacks
✓	✓	✓			Trails, lake views and farm animals
✓	✓			✓	Easy urban biking past farms and rivers
✓	✓	✓		✓	Bike on causeways across Lake Champlain
✓					Steep trail leads to amazing views
✓					Ridge-top hiking on Vermont's highest peak
✓		✓	✓		Loop hike to a fire tower
		✓ (paddle/swim)	✓		Wilderness paddling to island campsites
✓					Sweeping views from a ledgy summit
✓				✓	High-country hike to a craggy summit

PREFACE

There are few things we love more in this world than adventuring outdoors with our children, and we've found that northern New England is the perfect place to do it. Where else can families scour sandy beaches for hermit crabs, pick blueberries while hiking up forested and craggy mountains, get up-close-and-personal with farm animals, jump into crystal clear swimming holes at the base of waterfalls, bike along rolling hills, and paddle idyllic lakes or free-flowing streams…all in a summer weekend? Where else are the seasons so pronounced, providing different recreational opportunities every few months? Here, in northern New England, families' outdoor options are endless. Just when you start to think you can't handle summer's blackflies or winter's bitter cold, the season changes, transforming the landscape and presenting a whole new world of opportunity.

We wrote this book to share our love of New England's outdoors and because children today, more than ever, need encouragement to get outside. We've all heard the troubling statistic that children are spending half as much time outdoors as they did twenty years ago. As a result, physical fitness among kids is at an all-time low, while childhood obesity has more than doubled in the last 30 years. As the nature deficit grows, physical and psychological wellbeing is compromised. Studies demonstrate again and again how important direct contact with the outdoors is to healthy human development. Kids who play outside are generally stronger, healthier, and happier than their sedentary classmates.

By getting to know the natural world, children develop a sense of joy and wonder fundamental to living a good life. Just watch a child the first time she sees fireflies or looks out from a mountaintop at the vast view below: she can't help but drop her jaw and say, "Wow, that's awesome!" Her perspective shifts and she starts to recognize her place in a much larger world. New research suggests that this sense of awe, which makes us feel small and simultaneously connected to the world around us, is key to developing kids who are less self-absorbed and more engaged in meaningful, joyful, and compassionate ways of living.

We also wrote this book because we care about the future of the land and water, and we know the importance of developing tomorrow's conservation leaders. We met through the Student Conservation Association while leading teenagers on hands-on stewardship projects around the nation's public lands, and we saw again and again the light bulb go off in kids' heads when they recognized their role in the conservation movement. Getting kids outside at a young age is critical to fostering their environmental ethic. They must have direct experiences with nature in order to develop an emotional attachment to the environment. Only by caring will they commit to participating in environmentally friendly behaviors throughout their lives.

And, yes, we wrote this book because it was fun! It pushed us to revisit favorite destinations with a more discerning eye and venture out to new places that we might not otherwise have explored. Our kids are their happiest when given lots of space, so this project was as much for them as it was for us. They delighted in discovering the best swimming hole *ever*, the most awesome panoramic views, and the perfect paddling river. Sure, they complained at times, and things weren't always easy, but we did it together. We're stronger, healthier, happier families because we made it a priority to get outside. We unplugged our laptops and cell phones and got charged up by the natural world around us. It felt amazing. Go on, give it a try!

ACKNOWLEDGMENTS

This publication would not be possible were it not for our adventurous family and friends, to whom we dedicate this book. In particular, Ethan would like to thank his wife, Sarah, and their two children, Jackson and Tasha. Together, the Hipple family covered a lot of ground researching this book, and they did it with an inspiring sense of adventure. Yemaya would like to thank her husband, Lucas, and their two children, Gabriella and Waylon (who was in utero for much of the field work). Though the St.Clair kids are small, their love of the outdoors is huge. To all the friends who accompanied us on the trail, paddled and biked alongside us, shared notes and photos from the field, and encouraged us on this venture, we thank you. The Chamberlain-Kennedys, Deyessos, Albers, Tillman-Leddys, Clementses, Ellises, Baldwins, Caums, Peacock-Williamses, Beans, Reads, and Waldeier-Keeners deserve a special shout-out: your families make outdoor adventuring so much fun! We are both grateful to the Student Conservation Association for introducing us to and fostering our passion for environmental stewardship. We would also like to thank the Appalachian Mountain Club, and especially our editor, Victoria Sandbrook Flynn, who trusted us to make this book our own.

INTRODUCTION

For some, northern New England is synonymous with quaintness—Main Street, white-clapboard churches, maple syrup, covered bridges, red barns, historic brick buildings, and rural back roads. But this region, ripe for memory making, is also home to majestic granite mountains, rippling rivers, peaceful lakes, and so much more.

Maine, New Hampshire, and Vermont each have unique character and features. Politically, Maine straddles the bipartisan divide with an independent, "let everyone live for himself" attitude, while New Hampshire leans to the "don't tell me how to live" right and Vermont leans to the "let's all live peacefully together" left. Similarly, the states' landscapes are vastly different. Maine boasts arguably the nation's most spectacular coastline and forests while New Hampshire is known for its craggy peaks and Vermont for its open, rolling hills. Here are some unique characteristics of each three states.

Maine: This most northeastern state in the nation is one of the most sparsely populated and is nearly as large as the five other New England states combined. The immensity of its wilderness is difficult to comprehend. Maine's 32,000 miles of rivers and streams alone add up to more than the combined length of the Amazon, Nile, Yangtze, and Mississippi rivers.

Multiple recreational areas exemplify Maine's matchless landscapes. Acadia National Park in Downeast Maine is famous for its coastal beauty, but also includes majestic mountains, woodlands, and lakes. The park's Cadillac Mountain, accessible by foot or by vehicle, is the highest point along the North Atlantic seaboard. Bordering New Hampshire, the Western Lakes and Mountains region boasts some of the state's most scenic peaks and crystal clear bodies of water. The North Maine Woods is an impressive expanse of outstanding wilderness, including Baxter State Park with the 5,200-foot-tall Katahdin, the northern terminus of the Appalachian Trail. And then there is midcoast Maine with its plentiful sandy beaches and coastal hiking trails with spectacular views of the Atlantic Ocean.

Blueberries, lobster, and lighthouses are also synonymous with the state of Maine. In fact, Maine is the nation's largest producer of lowbush or "wild" blueberries and also the largest lobster producer, hauling in approximately 80 percent of the country's catch. Maine is also a mecca for lighthouses, with more than 60 along its craggy coastline.

New Hampshire: This fiercely independent state's nickname, "The Granite State," references its impressive granite formations and numerous quarries. When hikers think of New Hampshire, they usually think of the White Mountains—arguably the most rugged and spectacular range east of the Rockies. These truly spectacular peaks offer numerous summits that reach above treeline, and the surrounding White Mountain National Forest encompasses approximately 800,000 acres of land, 1,200 miles of trail, and countless lakes. It links the Vermont and Maine portions of the Appalachian Trail and is home to the Presidential Range with its 6,288-foot Mount Washington, the largest mountain in the Northeast and the site of the second highest recorded wind speed in the world. The Whites are also known for their system of eight high-alpine huts, operated by the Appalachian Mountain Club, which provide meals and lodging in a backcountry setting.

Farther north, New Hampshire's North Country is sometimes referred to as "north of the notches," referring to the White Mountain passes that channel traffic. This area is the state's least populated—a must-see for nature lovers on the search for wildlife, including moose, black bear, and deer.

The midstate Lakes Region is most famous for Lake Winnipesaukee, which is approximately 21 miles long and contains at least 253 islands. "Winnipesaukee" means either "smile of the Great Spirit" or "beautiful water in a high place," both of which speak to the fact that this is a particularly scenic area with excellent paddling opportunities. Unbeknownst to many, the Lakes Region actually harbors some "hidden" mountain ranges, most notably the Belknaps and the Ossipees, whose hidden hollows and crags beg to be explored.

To the southwest, the Sunapee region surrounds the popular Lake Sunapee while the Monadnock region traverses the highlands. Mount Monadnock itself is said to be the second most frequently climbed mountain in the world, after Japan's Mount Fuji. Along with several rocky summits, this region is studded with lakes, heath barrens, dense woodlands, and wetlands.

Farther southeast, the Merrimack Valley surrounds the Merrimack River, one of the larger waterways in New England. It empties into the Atlantic Ocean in Massachusetts; however, it is important to note that New Hampshire does, in fact, have an ocean coastline. At approximately 18 miles, it is the shortest ocean coastline of any state in the nation, and stands alone as the only state coastline that can be hiked in a day!

Vermont: Vermont is often shortchanged in regional guidebooks: it is the only landlocked state in New England and the nation's second least populous state and sixth smallest in terms of geographic area. While it is extremely rural—its valleys studded with farms and covered bridges—it is also extremely beautiful, rich with recreational opportunities.

The state is split east-west by the knobby spine of the Green Mountains. The 272-mile Long Trail, America's first (and some would say, best) long-distance hiking trail, traverses the high peaks of the Green Mountains and runs the length of the state. Vermont's nickname, "The Green Mountain State," speaks to its verdant hills and valleys, which are home to some of New England's greatest skiing, hiking, and biking. Vermont's unique geology also gives it some of the most phenomenal swimming holes in the country, which makes it a hit with kids of all ages. If you relish the thrill of finding that perfect emerald green pool with a sandy bottom and smooth granite slabs for sunning and jumping, this is your place.

One of the largest freshwater lakes in the nation, Lake Champlain is so big that it is said to have a mythical sea serpent. At 118 miles long and 12 miles across at its widest point, it hosts its own ferry system to shuttle cars between New York and Vermont, and even boasts the nation's only bike ferry. Like many of the state's other lakes and ponds, it is a treasured resource and important recreational area for swimming, boating, and fishing. The Champlain Valley offers incredible scenery, with hundreds of miles of hiking and biking trails interspersed with quaint New England villages and working family farms.

Vermont was once completely forested, but mankind has a way of altering natural landscapes. In the 1800s, approximately 80 percent of Vermont was cleared for pasture land. Today, only 25 percent remains open to pasture and farmland; the remaining 75 percent has reverted back to forest. In fact, only three states in the country have a higher percentage of forest than Vermont: West Virginia (77 percent), New Hampshire (78 percent), and Maine (85 percent)!

DISCOVERING YOUR FAMILY'S NORTHERN NEW ENGLAND

The recreational opportunities in northern New England are limitless, particularly for experienced hikers, bikers, and paddlers. Head any direction and you're likely to run into a mountain to climb, a river or lake to paddle, or a trail to bike. Knowing which ones aren't too steep, too fast, or too rough for your family, however, can be a challenge. In the next few sections, you'll find all the tips and tricks you'll need to get your family started in the great outdoors. When you're ready to start planning, select one of the trips in this book, which focuses exclusively on the best kid-friendly options, from stroller-friendly walks to calm waters to smooth rail-trails. Whether you live in northern New England or are just planning a visit, you'll find this book has what your family needs to get outside and enjoy the great outdoors.

HOW TO USE THIS BOOK

Planning an outdoor adventure with kids is different than planning one for adults. That is the guiding principle for this book. At first glance, it looks like any other recreational guidebook: the trip descriptions are organized geographically by state and then by region. But look closer!

To get an idea of which destination to choose, start with the regional locator map at the beginning of the book and the At-a-Glance Trip Planner. The chart summarizes the trips, giving you a snapshot of the destination and its features. Once you're ready to delve into one—or a few!—turn to the trip itself.

Beneath the trip name, a sentence or two highlights what makes this particular trip a must-do. Following that we've included all the necessary details:

- **Address:** If a particular street address isn't available, a street name and the two nearest intersections to the parking area or access point are given as well as the town.
- **Difficulty:** Trips are rated as easy, moderate, or challenging, depending on a number of factors such as distance, terrain, trail conditions, and elevation gain. Because this book includes destinations appropriate for kids up to age 12, some hikes are moderate or challenging. However, all paddling and biking trips are easy or easy-to-moderate. These ratings are all based on our opinions of the trips as authors and parents. Read each trip carefully and always take your own family's abilities into account!
- **Distance:** This lists either the one-way or round-trip distance in mileage. Paddling trips on lakes give round-trip distances with destinations like beaches and islands in mind. Note that many hiking trips' descriptions include optional turnaround points, so be sure to read the complete description before ruling out a hike as too long.
- **Hours:** If there are times (and/or particular months) when this destination is accessible, those will be listed here.
- **Fee:** Though many destinations are free to the public, some have use or parking fees. We recognize that fuel costs to remote destinations are expensive, so we've taken care to fill the book with free and low-cost trips.
- **Contact:** Here, we list the contact organization's name, phone number, and website (when each is available) where you can get additional up to date information. Note that hours, fees, and trail conditions are subject to

change, so it is always wise to check with the contact organization before heading out.

- **Bathrooms:** Some destinations have swanky restrooms, portable toilets, or outhouses. For others, a tree is your best option (see Stewardship and Conservation for Leave No Trace guidelines). Either way, you'll know what to expect before you arrive.
- **Water/Snacks:** If snack bars or water fountains are available on a trip, we'll list them here. Whether or not these amenities are available on-site, always bring your own snacks and water, just in case a food cart is closed or a fountain isn't running.
- **Maps:** While there are maps for some trips in this book, you should always review and bring reliable maps with you whenever possible, especially on backcountry trips. We've listed U.S. Geographical Survey topographical quadrants (USGS quads) as well as printed and digital maps where applicable and available.
- **Directions by Car:** Driving directions are given from the nearest city or large town. Parking information and global positioning system (GPS) coordinates are also included. While these coordinates entered into a GPS device will provide you with driving directions, we recommend always double-checking with an atlas like DeLorme's.

Read each trip's description thoroughly before setting out. Because this book includes destinations that are appropriate for kids up to age 12, some are more challenging than others and therefore not appropriate for small kids. On the flip side, some are more toddler-friendly, and might not sustain the interest of your pre-teen. Many trips offer optional turnaround points that make an otherwise challenging trip accessible for your family.

Unlike other guidebooks, we've emphasized Plan B options for each trip. Any number of factors can necessitate revising your plans, including inclement weather, forgotten gear, or even a change in attitude. But what really motivated us to expand the Plan B section was a recognition that kids love to mix things up. Sure, a hike might sound good in the morning, but what sounds *really* good is a splash in a crystal clear swimming hole at the heat of the day. "Better yet," we can hear our kids shouting, "let's do both!" Plus, with three states to cover—including an assortment of hikes, bikes, and paddles—we weren't able to include all of our favorite trips. Many of those that we reluctantly discarded on the cutting room floor are included here. They make great side trips to the main destinations or, in many cases, great trips on their own. While a destination hike or paddle may get you out of the house for the day or the weekend, we've found that some of our favorite family memories are made at places we find along the way: the roadside farm stand, the apple picking at the orchard down the road, or the hours spent lounging at the swimming hole.

The Nearby listing at the end of each trip notes where you can find nearby dining, lodging, shopping, or kid-friendly attractions such as children's museums or amusement parks—or the best local ice cream stand!

A photo or map accompanies each trip. Maps are always provided when necessary, particularly for loop hikes or bike rides with trail junctions. When photos are omitted, fear not: photos are available on kids.outdoors.org. This website is an excellent resource for updated information, and it offers you a platform where you, too, can share your notes from the field. We hope you do!

STEWARDSHIP AND CONSERVATION

Kids exploring nature experience an incredible sense of freedom. No walls exist. Social pressures to conform fall far from the trail. Kids can get dirty, make noise, and be their authentic selves. Yet, all freedoms come with responsibility. We must instill in our children a respect for the natural world to ensure that a healthy environment will be something all people can enjoy today and tomorrow.

The first step in encouraging children's conservation ethic is to foster their love for the outdoors. When they feel connected to a place—whether it is their neighborhood stream or their favorite mountain—they will recognize its value and understand the need to protect it. Even small children can have big feelings about the places they visit. Encourage them to share those feelings and describe what it is they love. Though it might be difficult for them to articulate, much of what they appreciate is likely nature's pure beauty. The lack of human interference on the landscape is what makes nature…well, natural. Sharing this perspective with kids will help them adopt the Leave No Trace guidelines described below.

Involving the whole family in stewardship activities is another great way to encourage a conservation-conscious child. Almost all environmental groups offer volunteer opportunities, many of which are appropriate for children. Activities might include picking up micro-trash at a public park, removing invasive species at a wetland, and even building trail features on a mountainside. The Appalachian Mountain Club (AMC) organizes many such stewardship opportunities, and the organization's regional chapters are a great resource for families. AMC programs get kids outdoors and teach conservation strategies through fun, hands-on experiences.

LEAVE NO TRACE

The Appalachian Mountain Club is a national educational partner of Leave No Trace, a nonprofit organization dedicated to promoting and inspiring responsible outdoor recreation through education, 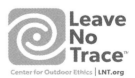 research, and partnerships. The Leave No Trace program seeks to develop wildland ethics—ways in which people think and act in the outdoors to minimize their impact on the areas they visit and to protect our natural resources for future enjoyment. Leave No Trace unites four federal land management agencies—the U.S. Forest Service, National Park Service, Bureau of Land Management, and U.S. Fish and Wildlife Service—with manufacturers, outdoor retailers, user groups, educators, organizations such as AMC, and individuals.

The Leave No Trace ethic is guided by these seven principles:

1. **Plan Ahead and Prepare.** Learn all you can about the area regulations before you head out. Be prepared; weather can change quickly and so can the temperature. Know where you are going, how you are going to get there, and make sure you tell at least one person of your itinerary.

2. **Travel and Camp on Durable Surfaces.** If you are hiking in a park area with hiking trails and established campsites then please use them. The purpose of designated hiking trails is to minimize the environmental damage to the area from hikers traipsing over the ground and ground cover.

3. **Dispose of Waste Properly.** Pack it in, pack it out. The best and easiest way to take your garbage out with you is to bring along a large Ziploc bag and toss your garbage inside. It stays sealed, it's waterproof, and you won't be leaving an unsightly mess for other hikers to see and the wildlife to deal with. Deposit solid human waste in cat holes dug 6 to 8 inches deep, at least 200 feet from water, camps, and trails. Pack out toilet paper and hygiene products. To wash yourself or your dishes, carry water 200 feet from streams or lakes and use small amounts of biodegradable soap. Scatter strained dishwater.

4. **Leave What You Find.** Sometimes it may be tempting to bring home a souvenir from your hiking trip. If everybody removed a souvenir or two what would be left for you to see? Digital cameras are great for capturing those memories. Cultural or historical artifacts, as well as natural objects such as plants and rocks, should be left as found.

5. **Minimize Campfire Impacts.** Cook on a stove. Use established fire rings, fire pans, or mound fires. Besides the danger of starting a forest fire, even small campfires can cause permanent damage to the surrounding area.

6. **Respect Wildlife.** Observe wildlife from a distance. Feeding the wildlife is hazardous to their health. They need to be able to hunt and find their own food without becoming reliant on hikers for snacks that may or may not be

part of their natural diet. Protect wildlife from your food by storing rations and trash securely.

7. **Be Considerate of Other Visitors.** Be courteous, respect the quality of other visitors' experience, and let nature's sounds prevail.

AMC is a national provider of the Leave No Trace Master Educator course. AMC offers this 5-day course, designed especially for outdoor professionals and land managers, as well as the shorter 2-day Leave No Trace Trainer course at locations throughout the Northeast.

For Leave No Trace information and materials, contact the Leave No Trace Center for Outdoor Ethics, P.O. Box 997, Boulder, CO 80306. Phone: 800-332-4100 or 302-442-8222; fax: 303-442-8217; web: lnt.org. For information on the AMC Leave No Trace courses, see outdoors.org/education/lnt.

GETTING STARTED

GETTING OUTSIDE NEAR HOME

Developing a love for the outdoors doesn't happen the first time a child camps in an iconic national park or climbs the peak of a majestic mountain. It happens over time, beginning with the seeds of natural wonder that are sown close to home. Children's comfort in the outdoors—as well as their confidence—grows with each successful outing, so it is important to set them up for success by starting small. For some families, this means setting a goal to get outside every day. That's all: get outside. For other families, it may mean increasing the time you spend outside daily or venturing beyond your backyard. But the backyard—whether it be a fenced-in grassy area or an empty city lot or your favorite park around the corner—is a great place to start.

Here are some activities that encourage kids to plug in to nature just about anywhere, any time of year:

- **Inside Out:** From board games to books, many traditional "indoor" activities can be set up outdoors, weather permitting. Once kids are appropriately dressed for the elements, they'll appreciate the change of scenery. They'll take comfort doing something familiar in an unfamiliar environment.
- **Treasure Hunt:** Create a list of natural objects you might find in your neighborhood and then head out on the hunt. Objects might include a fallen leaf, a rock, an insect, a pinecone, and a feather.
- **Sensory Walk:** Head out on a walk and touch, smell, look, and listen as you go. Try to awaken one sense at a time.
- **Fairy Land:** Gather together fallen natural objects such as twigs, pinecones, leaves, and rocks, then create mini houses for fairies or other favorite characters from your child's imagination.
- **Create-A-Fort:** Look for trees with branches that are low to the ground, bushes that are hollowed out in the middle, or logs, then create a fort around this base with fallen branches and tree boughs.
- **Night Watch:** Grab a flashlight and venture outside at night, taking in the transformed landscape and the starry night sky. Pay attention to the phase of the moon and keep an eye out for nocturnal wildlife.

In Every Season

Northern New England's pronounced seasons lend themselves well to season-specific outdoor activities. Here are some suggested ways to make the most of the seasons, without venturing far from home:

- **Fall:** Autumn is all about falling leaves, so go ahead, pile them up, toss them in the sky, and have a ball in fall. Bring a few leaves home to rub: just lay a leaf on a flat surface, cover it with white paper, rub the paper with a crayon, and watch the leaf shape emerge. Leaves can also be ironed between sheets of waxed paper to make bookmarks and window decorations.
- **Winter:** Bundle up and build a snowman, a snow fort, or a snow angel. Go sledding. Look for animal tracks (see Trip 70, Winter Adventures).
- **Spring:** New signs of life are everywhere! Look for buds on trees and flowers springing forth from the earth. Put on rain boots and splash in muddy puddles. Plant something and watch it grow. Easy-to-grow plants include sunflowers, lettuce, radishes, snow peas, and nasturtiums.
- **Summer:** Harvest vegetables right off the vine and pick berries at a local farm. Grab an inner tube and life jacket and float down a lazy river. Press flowers for craft projects. Catch insects and frogs. Live it up…it's summer!

GROWING UP OUTDOORS

Whether age 2 or 12, there are some things all children need to have successful outdoor adventures. Here's what you can do to help:

- **Share your enthusiasm:** When adults are truly excited about something, kids pick up on that energy and want to get in on the action.
- **Set up for success:** Plan an activity and trip that matches your child's interests and abilities. For example, if you know your child loves splashing in water, select a very short hike to a waterfall or swimming hole. Start small and close to home; build on those successes to venture farther afield.
- **Put safety first:** No matter their age, children require adult supervision, especially near water and on steep terrain. Pack the Ten Essentials (see later in this chapter), and be prepared to turn around whenever the conditions warrant.
- **Diversify the day:** Combining a hike with a short paddle and a dip in a swimming hole is a great way to keep your kids engaged outdoors all day.
- **Involve kids in the planning:** Kids love having a sense of control, so allow them to make certain choices. For example, they can decide between two trips you are considering, or choose what to include in the trail lunch. Greater ownership leads to fewer complaints.

- **Bring a friend:** Kids usually have more fun when they're with kids their own age, so consider inviting another child on your outing.
- **Rotate leaders:** When the way forward is clear, let kids lead. They'll pick up the pace and proudly advance the party when they're at the head of the line.
- **Praise, praise, praise:** Hiking, biking, and paddling aren't always easy, and kids efforts' need to be validated. Recognize when they're working hard, and tell them again and again what great explorers they are.
- **Pack snacks:** Along with a healthy trail lunch and plenty of water, pack a lot of different snacks. Consider including a few special treats that are not a part of your family's day-to-day diet.
- **Plan frequent stops:** Kids stop often, and sometimes they won't want to keep going. Use breaks wisely, refueling with snacks and water, taking in the natural environment, and preparing a trail game to keep everyone motivated (see Trip 21, Games On the Move).
- **Have patience:** There will be moments when you wish you'd just stayed home and plopped the kids in front of the TV. Remember, getting kids outdoors is highly rewarding in the long term. Whatever is making the experience less than enjoyable in the short term will change. We promise. Have patience.
- **Remember the big picture:** Don't feel bad about turning back, taking a shorter route, or not "accomplishing" something. Kids and parents should remember that the time they spend outdoors and together is always valuable.
- **Reward effort:** Often, a sweeping view or a perfect swimming hole is reward enough after physical exertion, but sometimes a special treat is in order. Consider finishing off your trip with a stop at a favorite café or ice cream stand. The adults probably deserve a cone as well!

Age-Specific Tips

Introducing your child to the outdoors with age-appropriate activities (and expectations) can help lay the groundwork for a great trip and many more to come!

Babies: We believe the earlier you introduce kids to the great outdoors, the better! As soon as you feel comfortable, snuggle your babe in a sling and head out to explore the neighborhood. Within a few months, your baby will be ready for the trail, tucked safely next to you in a front pack (check your child carrier's specifications for weight requirements). On boats, you can also hold infants in your lap or lay them right on the floor of the boat, where the rocking of the boat and the rhythmic paddling might put them right to sleep. It's not unrealistic to bring a 6 month old baby hiking or on a backcountry paddling trip as long as you are properly prepared and you know what you are getting into. As long as babies are fed, warm, and dry, they are generally good to go! Just note that babies aren't able to regulate their body temperatures the way older kids and adults do: check regularly to ensure that your baby isn't too hot or too cold. Also when paddling and biking, do not bring babies that are too small for infant life jackets and bicycle helmets.

Toddlers and Preschoolers: Toddling walkers are among the most curious—and slowest—outdoor adventurers. Prepare to move at a snail's pace, pausing often to check out critters and examine wildflowers and mushrooms. Children at this age do not have a long attention span, so plan accordingly. Even though the toddlers aren't babies anymore, this stage can actually be a more difficult time to go backpacking or on longer trips, so choose hikes that are less than a mile long, and prepare yourself to carry kids if necessary. When paddling and biking—both of which are activities that toddlers can't really do on their own—recognize that you'll still cover fewer miles because you're hauling a small person. Toddlers will best be stowed as passengers in the middle of a canoe or larger kayak. Help kids of this age stay engaged by singing silly songs and playing simple games. Be cognizant of toddlers' schedules: if naps are a normal part of your child's day, plan outings for before or after naptime.

Young Children (ages 5 to 8): In many ways, this age lends itself best to outdoor adventures: kids are physically coordinated and adventurous, while still focused more on their parents than their peers. They're eager to learn and discover new skills, and they're adept enough to help propel you forward on paddling and biking trips. On hiking trips, kids of this age can carry their own packs while walking up to 3 miles over easy-to-moderate terrain. Children in this age range can start tackling bike trips of 3 to 10 miles, round-trip. In boats, this age group can start to contribute to the paddling in either the middle or the bow (the "front") of the boat. An adult should always be in the stern (the "back") so they have the most control.

Older Children (ages 9 to 12): Keeping older children engaged is the name of the game, as kids this age need a good challenge to keep from getting bored. Relate a trip to your child's interests whenever you can. For example, if your child is into science, pack a field guide and magnifying glass or binoculars. If he's interested in art, bring a sketchpad and colored pencils. Physically fit kids will enjoy hikes that are moderate-to-challenging and include features such as waterfalls or steep terrain with hand-over-hand climbing. Mature kids might be ready to paddle their own canoe or pedal their bicycles farther than you'd expect (10 to 20 miles or more!). They'll definitely want to be involved in decision-making, so enlist their help with trip planning and navigation. Ask older kids to help with younger ones.

TRIP PLANNING

Creating successful trips with kids requires advanced planning. Select your destination carefully, taking into consideration the ages, physical fitness, coordination, and stamina of your children, as well as the season and weather forecast. When you're first starting off, choose shorter, easier trips than you think your kids can do; once you've gotten a feel for what your family likes and how far you can go, you can slowly increase distance and/or difficulty. Anytime you choose a destination, create a backup plan in case your first pick doesn't pan out—especially if you're planning an extended trip that requires a drive. Check the driving directions and parking information before heading out, and leave a copy of your itinerary with someone you trust. And don't forget to eat a good breakfast before leaving home!

Once you reach the trailhead or put-in location, take time to transition to the outdoors:

- Double check that you're carrying everything you intend to bring, including the Ten Essentials (see later in this section). There is nothing worse than forgetting your water or locking the keys in the car when you're far from help!
- Review the trip goals and route with your children. Remind them to stay together and always stop at junctions.
- Create a contingency plan just in case you get separated, the weather changes quickly, or the trip takes longer than you expected.
- Determine a turnaround time: you don't want to push your family to exhaustion or end up traveling unexpectedly in the dark, so make a plan and stick to it.
- Drink up! By starting a trip well hydrated, you'll get off on the right foot.
- Find the nearest bathroom or, if facilities aren't available, review the Leave No Trace guidelines for waste disposal.

The Ten Essentials

Bring the following items on *every* trip, no matter how close to home, no matter the forecast. Each one improves the chances that you are prepared for unexpected emergencies. Aside from food, water, and the specific map you'll need (which you'll add right before heading out), store these items together so you don't have to scramble to gather them every time you venture outdoors.

- **Navigation:** map and compass—and the knowledge to use them
- **Sun protection:** sunglasses, sunscreen, and sun hats
- **Insulation:** hat, gloves, socks, wool or synthetic sweater, and rain gear
- **Illumination:** headlamp or flashlight with extra batteries

- **First-aid supplies**: adhesive bandages, athletic or hospital tape, gauze, blister protection, small scissors, children's antihistamines, nonprescription painkillers, tweezers for removing splinters, and any important prescription medicine, including inhalers or an EpiPen if anyone in your party has severe allergies
- **Fire:** fire starter and matches or a lighter
- **Nutrition:** extra food that stores easily, such as high energy snacks like nuts, dried fruit, and granola bars
- **Hydration:** at least two quarts of water per person for day trips and a water filtration system if potable water is not available at the destination (if it is, it would be noted in the trip information)
- **Emergency shelter:** tarp or space blanket
- **Tools:** pocket knife or multitool and whistle

Along with the Ten Essentials, consider bringing these additional items to make your outing more comfortable and enjoyable:
- **Large plastic bags:** These have multiple functions, including pack liners to keep your gear dry, makeshift rain ponchos, trash bags, and emergency shelters.
- **Cell phone:** While a cellular phone can come in handy in emergencies, note that service is unreliable in rural and remote areas. Be cognizant of cell phone etiquette on the trail and use the phone only if absolutely necessary.
- **Insect repellent:** During summer when blackflies and mosquitoes are abundant, having repellent on hand is necessary. Do not apply DEET on babies' skin, and use it sparingly on young children, avoiding their hands, eyes, and mouth area.
- **Bandana, handkerchief, or wet wipes:** Kids get bumps, scrapes, and snotty noses indoors and out, and sometimes the very best remedy is a good old piece of cloth.
- **Binoculars, field guides, journal, bug net, magnifying glass:** Natural history will come to life with a few extra resources like these.
- **Camera:** Capture your family's outdoor adventures.
- **Umbrellas:** While some backcountry enthusiasts may scoff at bringing an umbrella ("we have rain gear instead!"), an umbrella is a remarkably useful outdoors device. It can create a lightweight, portable, instant shelter—anywhere you want it! We bring them for short day hikes or the longest multi-week expeditions. You still need to bring your rain gear and shell layers, but the addition of an umbrella will keep everyone much drier and happier.

Outdoors with Kids Basics

When you're enjoying a hike or a paddle on your own, you may actually *avoid* the easy routes, but with kids, try to keep everything as simple and easy as possible. Whether it's your first time trying these activities or you're just starting to think about sharing your love for the outdoors with your kids, you'll need to plan your trips a bit differently than when you head out on your own.

- **Hiking:** If you have a choice, always ascend steep sections and descend gradual sections, as it is easier on your body and safer as well.
- **Biking:** Start your bike trip at a lower elevation, so that you are working hardest at the beginning of the day, and can coast home when you are tired!
- **Paddling:** Lake paddling is best for families new to paddling, and you can spend hours exploring secluded bays and inlets. Our kids like to think of rivers as "nature's conveyor belts" because at times you can just sit there and enjoy the view as the river carries you downstream. Start early, especially on large lakes. While day-to-day weather patterns will change, winds tend to whip up larger waves in the afternoon on large lakes like Umbagog, Champlain, and Winnipesaukee.

Swimming Hole Safety and Etiquette

We have highlighted many swimming holes in this book and we hope that your families will enjoy them as much as we do! Nothing beats discovering an emerald green pool with a sandy bottom after a hike on a humid day. To keep these special places clean and safe for everyone, please follow these general guidelines, and encourage others you see to do so as well.

Nothing ruins a swimming hole more than trash left behind. Remember your Leave No Trace ethics and leave the place better than you found it. Bring a small plastic bag to pick up any trash left by others.

Never jump into a swimming hole without testing the depth first. Ease in from the beach or the bank, swimming to the spot to which you plan to jump, and test the depth by swimming to the bottom.

Currents can be strong any time of year, but particularly in spring or after a heavy rainfall. Never swim in flood-stage waters or in currents that will carry you downstream.

Leave anything made of glass at home. Glass bottles can break and injure people and animals.

Most swimming holes don't have bathroom facilities. If you must relieve yourself, do so at least 200 feet from the water, digging a cat hole at least 6 inches deep and covering it up afterward (see Leave No Trace).

Bring a warm layer to throw on afterward. New England brooks are notoriously cold, so even on a hot day throwing on a hoodie or a nice fuzzy fleece afterward feels good!

Bike Trail Etiquette
- Be considerate of other trail users.
- Only stray from the trail on public areas.
- When stopping on the trail, move off the traveled portion of the trail if you can, or as far to the right as possible.
- Keep pets on leash and clean up after them.
- When passing horses (which are allowed in some trail sections), use a calm voice.
- Bikes yield to walkers and horses.
- Walkers yield to horses.
- Riders always wear a helmet! Set a good example for your kids!
- Always ride slowly in single file when meeting others or being overtaken.
- Ride in a straight line. This is especially difficult for children, so remind and encourage them not to weave around on the trail.
- When overtaking other trail users, call out a warning, such as "passing on your left" or use a warning device such as a bell. Be especially careful when passing children.
- Share the trail with wildlife.
- During hunting season, wear orange blaze.

Camping
Camping at campgrounds or "car camping" is a great way to combine several trips into a multiday adventure. We have listed convenient campgrounds near many of the trips, but don't be constrained by these options; all three states covered in this book have excellent state park systems with clean, well-tended campgrounds, and National Forest campgrounds are excellent as well.

Backpacking with infants is possible as long as you have a few adults to help split the load: one parent will need to carry the baby and a smaller amount of gear. Backpacking with toddlers is virtually impossible, as they are too big to carry for any length and too small to carry a pack or hike very far. Once kids reach 7 to 10, they are ready to hoist a pack and carry their share of gear to reach magical backcountry destinations! We have listed several options in this book that make excellent first backpacking trips as they are within a couple miles of the trailhead, but still offer the thrill of a backcountry camping experience.

Canoe and kayak camping with kids is surprisingly easy—and unlike back packing, you can bring toddlers and infants along for the ride! For those of you longing to get into remote backcountry with young kids, there is no better way to do it than in a canoe or kayak. You can bring along more supplies and better food in your boat than you can fit in a backpack, which makes it a great way to introduce kids to the wonders of backcountry travel. It is a much easier way to get into remote places than backpacking, so the kids can focus on the positive and fun parts of wilderness travel instead of the grueling marches uphill with heavy packs on their backs.

OUTDOOR CLOTHING AND GEAR

Whether hiking, biking, or paddling, follow these basic rules for what to wear:

- **Avoid cotton:** When cotton gets wet, it stays wet. While a cotton T shirt is fine for a short midsummer outing, choose synthetic materials when possible. While high-tech clothing can be expensive, you can often find it reasonably priced at thrift stores or gear swaps.
- **Layer up:** Dress in a number of lightweight clothes that you can add or remove in response to changing conditions and your various level of activity. This is especially important fall through spring! The thin, wicking base layer goes on first, next to the skin. Then comes the mid-layer, which could be lightweight wool or nylon. The insulating layer that follows is designed specifically to provide warmth; appropriate materials include fleece, pile, and wool. The outer layer is the final layer, consisting of tops and bottoms that protect you from wind and weather. The layering system takes some getting used to, so kids will need lots of help adjusting their layers to fit their needs and the environment.
- **Go long:** Long-sleeved shirts and long pants protect skin from sun, bugs, thorny bushes, and poisonous plants.
- **Choose appropriate footwear:** Socks and closed-toe shoes are a must. Whenever possible, wear shoes that have already been broken in to avoid blister care on-the-go.
- **Comfort is key:** Make sure clothing and footwear fits properly and feels good.

Keep the above rules in mind no matter what activity you choose, and read on for clothing and gear information specific to hiking, biking, paddling, and camping.

Hiking

Appropriate footwear is especially important when hiking. Along with being closed-toe and comfortable, hiking boots should be lightweight with sturdy soles, good ankle support, and moisture-resistance. Sneakers may be adequate for easy hikes over level terrain, while boots are necessary for anything moderate to difficult. In winter and during mud season, boots are a must.

Carry a backpack to hold your Ten Essentials and additional items. Backpacks should be lightweight but sturdy, with a waist belt to help distribute the load. Pack lightly, keeping in mind that you may end up carrying your child at times. Encourage kids over 4 years old to carry their own small packs, but oversee their contents. The last thing you want is to end up carrying your backpack, your child, his backpack, and all the stuffed animals and toys he crammed inside!

Carry babies and young toddlers in child carriers. The range of carriers today can be overwhelming, so when deciding which to use, follow these guidelines:

- A newborn should be carried in a simple, frameless infant carrier pack that snuggles your baby right in front of you.
- After babies develop head control and can sit up on their own, transition to a child carrier with built-in frame that holds the child upright behind you. Features should include adjustable shoulder and waist straps and an adjustable child harness.
- Parental comfort is key, so get help adjusting a pack to fit your body before heading out on the trail.
- Though many external frame child carriers have kickstands that provide a stable platform for loading and unloading your child, note that kids should never be left unattended while in their carriers.

Biking

Young kids don't need to be able to pedal to enjoy a good bike trip, but they do need to sit up on their own and fully support their head before they can snuggle into a carrier and come along for the ride. When dressing for bike rides, follow the clothing guidelines for hiking, with one exception: if children are pedaling, they should wear shorts or make sure the bottoms of their pants are tucked into their socks to ensure they don't get snarled in the chain.

Attached bike seats and trailers are both viable options for toddlers. Most bike seats are suitable for children weighing up to 40 pounds, and some parents prefer them because kids are highly visible to others and less exposed to car exhaust. It is important to note, however, that the child will fall if the adult falls. With bike trailers, on the other hand, your child won't fall even if you do, and trailers can haul kids up to 6 years old.

When kids are ready to branch off, get them started with a push bike, balance bike, or training wheel bike. A push or balance bike—which has neither pedals nor a chain—helps 2 to 5 year olds coordinate their steering and balance. Bikes with training wheels can give children the confidence they need to start riding on their own, when training wheels are removed. Trailer bikes are another great option: they allow children to pedal and feel independent while still relying on adults for balance and control. Trailer bikes attach to the back of adult bikes and are good for 4- to 7-year-olds. They allow adults to cycle farther than they might otherwise be able to with kids in tow. Children with good balance and coordination can graduate to their own 2-wheeler. Most of the bicycle trips included in this book are appropriate for mountain bikes or hybrid bikes with knobby tires, which can handle the gravel and dirt trails.

Whether riding in a trailer, in a bike seat, or on a bike, a brand new, well-fitted helmet is a must. The earlier a child gets comfortable wearing a helmet, the better. Helmet retailers should be able to assist you with correct fit.

Paddling

When paddling, children should always wear personal flotation devices (PFDs) as most state laws require. Parents should set an example by wearing PFDs as well. PFDs come in five types. Most children will use a Type III, which is a flotation aid suitable for various activities. Infants can use Type II PFDs, which are designed for use in calm waters. Ensure the PFD fits your child well. The PFD should fit snugly. Choose based on your child's weight:

- Infant PFDs are for children 8 pounds to 30 pounds
- Child PFDs are for children 30 pounds to 50 pounds
- Youth PFDs are for children 50 pounds to 90 pounds

To test the fit, secure your child in the PFD, then grasp the shoulders of the PFD and lift your child. His or her ears and chin should not slip through the PFD.

When paddling, store gear in specialized dry bags or in double-bagged, heavy-duty plastic bags. You can make a low-cost dry bag by simply putting one or two 2.5-mm trash compactor bags inside of a nylon stuff sack and twisting it shut. Older children can be responsible for their own bags of personal gear.

Camping

Camping with kids can be a challenge: you have to bring more gear than you do on a trip with just adults. This can make backpacking particularly challenging, but car camping and overnights with boats offer more flexibility for packing more gear. Besides the Ten Essentials, bring these items if you can:

- **Games and activities:** Bring along a deck of cards, dice, and paper and pencil to play some games by the fire. Bring along the fishing rod, bikes, arts and crafts books. Leave the iPods, tablets, and phones at home.
- **Great food:** Meals can be the high point of a camping trip and are a great morale booster, especially when it is cold or wet. We even bring the cast-iron Dutch oven when we car and canoe camp to make lasagna, pizzas, and sticky buns!
- **Extra sleeping bags:** Having an extra sleeping bag (especially on a back-country trip) can help when someone has an accident, gets sick in their bag, or just needs some extra warmth.

Your shelter matters a great deal when you're planning to spend the night out. Bring everything it takes to set it up and secure it against the elements. Make sure you have all of your tent poles and stakes before you leave home. Set your rain fly secure and tight, or it just simply won't work and you will have some unhappy campers. Make sure you don't set up your tent in a low spot where water will collect when it rains. Wet kids are unhappy kids.

Winter Fun

Avoid cabin fever during the long New England winters by getting outside. These tips will help you stay warm and dry as you take advantage of the winter wonderland:

- Dress children in multiple layers—including warm, insulating pieces. Remember that active people (including kids) generate heat quickly, so help them remove layers as necessary.
- One-piece snowsuits work best for younger children. Older children should practice the same layering system as adults.
- Balaclavas are great winter hats for kids because they cover both head and neck, leaving just an opening for the face.
- Keep toes warm—invest in a pair of wool or fleece socks.
- Mittens keep hands warmer than gloves, so unless children need to use their fingers, mittens are best in winter. Wool socks can double as mittens.
- Remember sunglasses when out on the snow.
- Bring packets of hand warmers and foot warmers for emergencies (like "I forgot my gloves"); they're inexpensive and long-lasting, and they can make all the difference to the success of an outing on a cold day.
- Select snowshoes by weight of the wearer, and look for ones that are easy for children to put on and take off.

- Waxless skis are the best choice for children who are learning the basics of cross-country skiing.
- Many Nordic centers and downhill ski resorts rent snowshoes and cross-country ski equipment for children.
- When cross-country skiing, it's easier and safer to use a sled built specifically for pulling children, called a pulk, than it is to ski with a baby in a backpack or front child carrier. You may start using a pulk with a child between 6 and 12 months old. The sled has two poles that are secured to the adult with a padded waist belt. Many cross-country ski areas have pulks available for rent.
- Warm liquids are a welcome comfort in the cold: fill a thermos with hot chocolate or your family's favorite soup and pack it along.

SAFETY

Outdoor activities involve inherent risk, most of which can be managed with proper foresight and preparation. First and foremost it is important to recognize your own strengths and limitations, and those of the rest of the group. Traveling anywhere with kids means completely altering your expectations: let the physical and developmental abilities (or lack thereof) of your youngest child be your guide. If you question whether a particular trip is within a child's abilities, err on the side of caution.

Children often become so engrossed in an activity that they ignore discomfort until it becomes unbearable. It's as if a switch flips, and suddenly they're miserable (and possibly in danger). Anticipate your child's needs and plan accordingly. There are a number of environmental concerns that can become issues when not immediately addressed, no matter how easy or difficult the terrain and activity:

Inclement Weather

Check the forecast before heading out and be prepared to change course at any point if the weather turns. Mountain ranges often have their own weather systems that don't show up on the forecast of your local news station. The higher the elevation, the more extreme the weather is likely to be. Northern New England is known for its ferocious storms; you don't want to try navigating through one with your children.

Sun and Heat

Maine, New Hampshire, and Vermont may be far from the equator, but the sun's force can still be mighty. During very hot weather, choose activities in the shade or close to water where kids can quickly cool off. Make sure children are dressed appropriately and drinking enough water. Doing so will help prevent heat exhaustion or heat stroke, both of which have symptoms that include headache, dizziness, pale skin, nausea, and shallow breathing. If a child becomes overheated, move them to a cool, shady spot; loosen clothing; apply wet cloths; and encourage small sips of water.

Avoid sunburns by applying sunscreen thoroughly at least 30 minutes before exposure and every two hours after that. Babies under 6 months should not be exposed to direct sun, as their skin is extremely sensitive to the sun's rays and to the chemical ingredients in sunscreen.

Hypothermia

Hypothermia is a medical emergency resulting from dangerously low body temperature. Because children lose heat more quickly than adults, it's critical to be aware of the signs and symptoms, as well as the conditions during which hypothermia is possible. It can happen in any season, particularly in cool, wet, windy weather, as well as in colder, drier conditions. Prevent hypothermia by dressing warmly in layers, and by staying dry, well hydrated, and nourished.

Keep an eye out for early signs of hypothermia, when a child becomes cranky and listless and complains of being cold. Signs of more advanced hypothermia include shivering, stumbling, sleepiness, decreased motor skills, loss of judgment, and impaired speech (including slurred words). Check babies and young children often; if their neck, torso, or limbs feel cool to the touch, add layers and seek shelter. If any child becomes chilled, remove her from the cold, wet conditions; change her into dry, warm clothing; wrap her in a sleeping bag or other insulating material; and encourage her to sip warm, sweet liquids and eat food with protein and sugar.

Dehydration

Kids rarely drink enough water when active outdoors, unless an adult reminds them to do so. Dehydration is especially likely to happen in hot weather, direct sunlight, or when sweating hard. Watch out for the signs of dehydration, which include dry mouth, dark yellow urine (or less urine than usual), irritability, and lightheadedness. Treat mild dehydration by slowly trying to replace fluids. Remove kids from the heat and get them to rest until they are rehydrated.

The best way to ensure you have plenty of potable water is to bring it with you. Never drink untreated water from an unknown source. If backcountry camping, always bring a water-filtration system, an iodine-based disinfectant, or the equipment you need to boil water.

Insects

While mosquitoes and blackflies can be annoying, the potentially dangerous insect to guard against is the nearly microscopic deer tick. These tiny parasitic creatures can spread Lyme disease, a potentially serious illness that can lead to neurological disorders. By taking preventive measures to guard against ticks, you'll also guard against mosquitoes and blackflies.

Dress children in long sleeves, long pants, and light colored clothing so that it's easier to spot ticks. Tuck pants into socks, protecting feet and ankles while preventing ticks from crawling underneath clothing. Apply insect repellent to clothing and exposed skin, but note that repellent containing DEET is not recommended for children. At the conclusion of a trip, do a family "tick check," paying close attention to the areas inside and behind the ears, along the hairline, at the back of the neck, between toes, behind knees, and in armpits and groin. If you find a tick on your child, remove it as soon as possible (visit cdc.gov/ticks for tips).

Poisonous Plants

Children should learn to not touch plants or eat berries before first asking an adult. Poison ivy is pervasive in northern New England, particularly in disturbed areas, roadsides, and the edges of fields. The oil in its leaves, vines, and roots causes an allergic reaction. Teach kids the following rhyme to help them identify and steer clear of poison ivy: "Leaves of three, let them be. If it's hairy, it's a berry; if it's shiny, watch your hiney." If children come in contact with poison ivy, wash the affected area with soap and cold water as soon as possible.

There are many trips in this book with blueberries you can enjoy. If you choose to let your children partake in the summer feast, monitor them carefully. Older children can learn how to safely identify common wild edible fruits and berries; local nature centers are a good source of educational programs.

Animals

Teach children to observe, but not feed, wild animals. Explain that they shouldn't get between a mother and her young, such as a mother bear and cubs or a moose cow and calves. If you are camping in the backcountry, always use a canister to ensure that your food, drinks, and toiletries don't attract wildlife.

Lightning

Thunderstorms are common in New England, and all thunderstorms produce lightning, which is dangerous. Watch the sky, looking for darkening skies, flashes of lightning, or increasing winds. If you hear thunder, immediately seek shelter in a sturdy building or car. If neither is available, crouch down in an open area, staying twice as far away from a tree as it is tall. Alternately, seek shelter among a stand of trees that are of equal height. Avoid metal, drop backpacks and trekking poles, and stay out of water. If you are paddling and see a storm approaching, immediately head for shore. Wait at least 30 minutes after the last observed lightning strike or roll of thunder before resuming activity.

Water Safety

Kids need constant supervision around water, even if they know how to swim. Invest in proper fitting, Coast Guard-approved PFDs (see Outdoor Clothing and Gear: Paddling) and make sure they are well fitted to your child. For kids younger than 5 years old, choose life jackets with head support and a strap between the legs. The Coast Guard cautions that Infant Type II personal flotation devices up to 18 pounds may not always perform as expected. Create a water safety culture in your family so that kids know to always wear their life jackets and to approach water only with adult supervision. Know how to safely operate any watercraft you use before bringing children aboard. Establish rules for your family and enforce them without fail (for example, no swimming unless you can touch bottom).

Getting Lost

The best way to avoid getting lost is to stay found. Kids should learn to stick with the group, stay on the trail, and wait at trail junctions for *everyone* to catch up. If there is one rule of thumb to keep from getting lost, it is to *wait at every trail intersection* for all hikers! Enforce this vigilantly so that kids learn this early on and it just becomes a habit. New England hiking trails are often marked with blazes and rock cairns: make sure you can always see one blaze ahead and one behind. Help orient kids to their surroundings by pointing out landmarks along the way. Teaching children map and compass skills is a great idea, as is enrolling in an orienteering or survival program such as those offered through AMC.

Teach your children what to do if they become separated from the group: stay in one place (preferably in the open); blow three short blasts on your whistle; make a return noise if you hear a noise (which could signal someone is looking for you); and do your best to stay calm.

Section 1

Coastal Maine

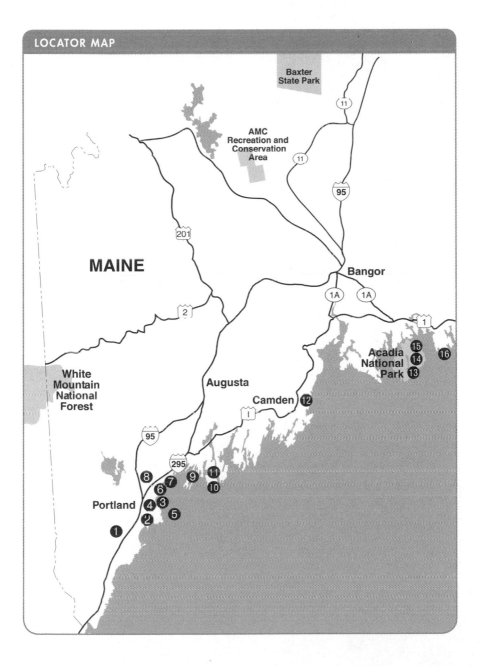

LOCATOR MAP

Baxter State Park

AMC Recreation and Conservation Area

MAINE

Bangor

Acadia National Park

White Mountain National Forest

Augusta

Camden

Portland

Trip 1

Ages 5+

Scarborough Marsh Audubon Center

Explore Maine's largest saltwater marsh and get up-close-and-personal with a dazzling array of wildlife.

Address: 136 Pine Point Road, Scarborough
Difficulty: Easy–Moderate
Distance: 2.6–8.0 miles, round-trip
Hours: 9:30 A.M.–5:30 P.M., June–Labor Day and special occasions
Fee: Free; canoe and kayak rentals available
Contact: 207-883-5100, maineaudubon.org/find-us/scarborough-marsh
Bathrooms: At the Nature Center
Water/Snacks: Water fountain at the nature center; snacks at the nature store
Maps: USGS Cumberland County quad; *Maine Atlas and Gazetteer*, Map 3: B3 (DeLorme)
Directions by Car: From US 1 in Scarborough, turn east onto Pine Point Road/ ME 9. Turn left into the Nature Center parking in 0.8 mile (43° 33.238′ N, 70° 29.099′ W).

The Scarborough Marsh estuary boasts the state's largest salt marsh and excellent paddling opportunities that get you up-close-and-personal with a dazzling array of wildlife. When you arrive, take the time to explore the Nature Center, which features exhibits, a nature store, walking trails, and canoe rentals, as well as knowledgeable volunteers who will help guide you toward the estuary's best features.

Rent kayaks or canoes in season, or launch your own. Because the Nature Center and boat launch are located approximately in the middle of the 2,700 acres of marsh, you can choose to head inland or toward the sea. There are two things to take into consideration when making your choice—the tide and the current. Paddling against the tide on the leg out, when you have the most energy, is a good idea as the tide and current will help you return on the leg back. Keep in mind that paddling toward the sea will take you into waters with stronger current and potentially some chop. The distance from the Nature Center to the mouth of the harbor is approximately 4 miles. For a shorter

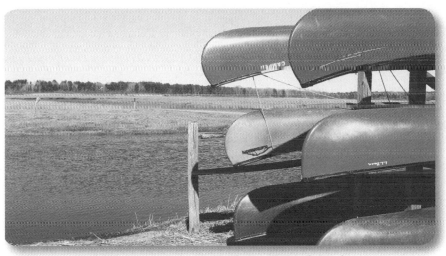

*Bring your own canoe or kayak to Scarborough Marsh
or rent one, in season, at the Nature Center.*

paddle, turn around at the bridge to the Eastern Trail (Trip 2), which is 1.3 miles from the Nature Center.

Paddling inland offers more protection. Unless you and your children are skilled paddlers, stay inland. Head toward Route 1, which is approximately a 2-mile paddle from the Nature Center. The marsh's multiple small channels give the estuary a maze-like quality that children love. The more narrow the channel, however, the more likely it will dead-end. Stick to wider channels if you want to avoid backtracking.

Encourage children to have some quiet time along the route to fully experience this rich ecosystem. An amazing array of wildlife depends on this habitat for food and shelter, including egrets, herons, glossy ibises, muskrats, minks, and otters. The quieter and more still you can be, the higher the likelihood you will spot an animal you have never seen before.

While the opportunities for exploring the marsh seem limitless, eventually it will be time to turn your boat around and return to the center. Whether you choose to head toward sea or stay inland, remain mindful of the tides, and plan your return trip accordingly.

PLAN B: Consider stretching your legs on the self-guided nature trail that leaves from the back deck of the Nature Center. Pick up a detailed brochure, which provides natural history information corresponding with the eleven marked stations along the trail. Find additional nearby walking and biking opportunities along the Eastern Trail (Trip 2).

NEARBY: For a bite to eat, head back to US 1 in Scarborough.

Trip 2

All Ages

Eastern Trail

Flat, off-road terrain through mixed forest and salt marsh makes this the perfect destination for wheels, whether you're on bikes, in a wheelchair, or pushing a stroller.

Address: Black Point Road and Eastern Road, Scarborough
Difficulty: Easy–Moderate
Distance: 16.8 miles, round-trip
Hours: Sunrise to sunset
Fee: Free
Contact: Eastern Trail Alliance, 207-284-9260, easterntrail.org
Bathrooms: Portable toilet on the trail
Water/Snacks: None
Maps: USGS Prouts Neck and Old Orchard Beach quads; easterntrail.org/index. php/trails-a-maps
Directions by Car: From I-295, Exit 2, take US 1 south. Merge onto Scarborough Connector and then continue onto ME 9 W/US 1 S. Travel 1.2 miles and turn left onto Black Point Road, then right onto Eastern Road. Travel to the end of the road to access the ample parking area and trailhead (43° 34.903′ N, 70° 20.303′ W).

The East Coast Greenway is a developing trail that will one day wind its way from northern Maine to Key West, Florida, linking all the major cities of the eastern seaboard on safe, traffic-free paths. Parts of that trail are already established, including Maine's Eastern Trail, which currently spans a scenic 65-mile signed bike route from the Piscataqua River in Kittery northward to Casco Bay in South Portland. The Eastern Trail Alliance's maps are geo-tagged with various points of interest, allowing users to plan where on their cycling trips they'll pause to take in vistas or stop for a bite to eat. Though some of the trail is on paved road, off-road sections are plentiful and expanding annually. The most kid-friendly section of the trail is this 8.4-mile off-road stretch from Scarborough to Saco. While street crossings along the trail are well marked with crosswalks and ample signage, take extra caution: many cars and trucks speed along these backcountry roads and aren't prepared to stop quickly for crossing bikers and pedestrians. Prior to setting off on the trail, warn your

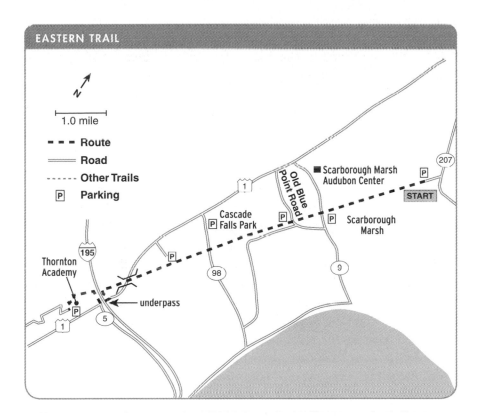

children about the road crossings and set expectations for crossing together as a group once adults have determined it is safe to do so.

A kiosk near the Scarborough trailhead provides information about the trail system, as well as tips for good trail etiquette. The wide trail is primarily composed of compacted, crushed gravel, which makes for pleasant, easy riding terrain. In the late 1800s, this surprisingly straight trail was a rail corridor for the Eastern Railroad that connected Maine with Boston. Since the rail line was removed at the end of World War II, this old corridor became overgrown and forgotten before it became a natural gas corridor and, more recently, a celebrated recreation trail.

The first mile of trail cuts through mixed forest before opening onto the 2,700-acre Scarborough Marsh (see Trip 1), Maine's largest salt marsh and home to abundant bird species and other wildlife. A wide, modern bridge leads over the water and continues through the marsh before crossing Pine Point Road and ducking back into the woods.

The trail continues through mixed forest dotted with occasional benches along the way. At approximately 7.0 miles, the trail crosses over US 1 via the John Andrews Bridge. Soon thereafter, it turns sharply to the left (south) and leads through an I-195 underpass. Access to and from the underpass is relatively steep, and children may need to dismount and walk their bicycles through this short section. The trail straightens again before ending in Saco at Thornton Academy (8.4 miles), which is near the former Portland airport where Charles Lindbergh frequently landed. To return to the Scarborough trailhead off Eastern Road, turn around here.

PLAN B: Another popular segment of the Eastern Trail is the 5.7-mile section from Bug Light Park in Portland to Highland Avenue in South Portland (also known as the South Portland Greenbelt). This trail offers a more urban route, some of which is on asphalt. To reach Bug Light from I-295, Exit 6A, follow State Route 77 across the Casco Bay Bridge. Continue straight (don't follow Route 77) on Broadway to the T junction, turn left on Breakwater Drive and then turn right on Madison Street. Follow signs for the lighthouse to the large parking lot, which is the launching point for Bug Light Park's many trails. The park was once home to the Portland Shipyard where hundreds of Liberty Ships were produced for World War II. Here at the park, look for passing sailboats, ferries and tankers, and take a moment to enjoy Bug Light, the lighthouse at the tip of the breakwater. Eastern Trail signs mark the beginning of the route, which links residential areas, schools, parks, recreation centers, retail areas, and marinas.

NEARBY: Both Scarborough and Saco offer plenty of dining options. In Scarborough, look for markets and restaurants along US 1. In Saco, Main Street offers many dining options, as well as a historic walking tour.

Trip 3

Back Cove and Eastern Promenade Trails

This off-road, family-friendly trail is perfect for biking, offering great views of Portland's skyline and idyllic waterfront.

Address: Preble Street (between Baxter Boulevard and Marginal Way), Portland
Difficulty: Easy–Moderate
Distance: 7.7 miles, round-trip
Hours: Dawn to dusk
Fee: Free
Contact: Portland Trails, 207-775-2411, trails.org/our-trails
Bathrooms: Portable toilets at Edward Payson Park; restrooms at East End Beach
Water/Snacks: None
Maps: USGS Portland West and Portland East quads; trails.org/our-trails
Directions by Car: From I-295, Exit 6B, take US 302/ME 100/Forest Avenue west and take the next right on Baxter Boulevard. In 0.1 mile, turn right on Preble Street and park in the large public parking lot on your left, across the street from the Hannaford grocery store (43° 39.909′ N, 70° 16.078′ W).

The two trails described here, when combined, make for an excellent bike route that even beginners will enjoy. With plenty of rest stops along the way, picturesque views, and kid-friendly attractions (Did someone say sandy beach? Dog park? Playground? Train museum?), it's no wonder these wide, flat trails are Portland's most popular havens for bikers, joggers, and dog-walkers. Be prepared to share the trail.

From the Back Cove parking lot, head west on the path at the north end of the lot. It quickly merges onto Baxter Boulevard Path, which has trail markers every 0.25 mile and occasional benches. Looking back over the bay, which drains at low tide, enjoy wide spanning vistas of the Portland skyline as you make your way around Back Cove. At approximately 2.0 miles, the path reaches Edward Payson Park on your left, an excellent pit stop if you're looking for bathrooms or a break from pedaling. The park includes a playground, tennis courts, playing fields, and even a wintertime terrain park.

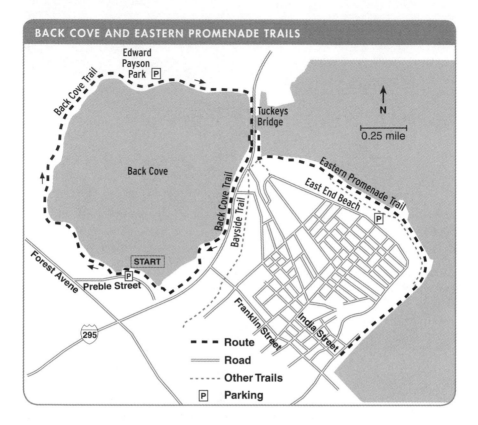

BACK COVE AND EASTERN PROMENADE TRAILS

Edward Payson Park

Back Cove Trail

Tuckeys Bridge

N

0.25 mile

Back Cove

Eastern Promenade Trail

East End Beach

Back Cove Trail

Bayside Trail

START

Forest Avene

Preble Street

Franklin Street

India Street

295

- - - Route

Road

- - - - - Other Trails

P Parking

Back on the bike, continue pedaling around the north end of Back Cove to Tukey's Bridge, which connects the Portland peninsula to East Deering across the cove. Here, stay on the bike path, proceeding slowly under the bridge. This is the trickiest part of the ride, as the trail is narrow, curved, and congested with other bikers and pedestrians. Fortunately, it's a short stretch. Within a few hundred feet the path merges onto well-marked 2.1-mile Eastern Promenade Trail (known locally as the East End Trail) to continue to Portland's Old Port. The trail is paved and scenic, skirting the perimeter of Casco Bay while offering stunning ocean vistas. Consider stopping to get your feet wet at the small and sandy East End Beach, Portland's only public beach. (Public restrooms and changing areas are available at the nearby boat launch.) Offshore, you'll see sailboats bobbing on their moorings and islands that beckon, including Peaks Island (Trip 5), Great Diamond Island, and Long Island. Near the terminus of the trail, notice the defunct rail cars and the restored passenger trail of the Maine Narrow Gauge Railroad Co. & Museum, which offers 40-minute train rides along the Eastern Promenade Trail from May through October (mainenarrowgauge.org).

The Eastern Promenade Trail ends at the eastern edge of Portland's Old Port (3.75 miles), at the corner of Commercial and India streets. If you have the time and inclination, consider exploring the Old Port restaurants and shops before turning around and retracing the path to Tukey's Bridge. Once under the bridge, merge with Back Cove Trail and pedal along the western edge of Back Cove until returning to the parking lot where you began.

PLAN B: For a shorter option, consider completing just one of the two sections of trail. Back Cove Trail, by itself, is a 3.5-mile loop. The Eastern Prom Trail is 2.1 miles, one-way; reach its trailhead near the eastern end of Portland's Old Port, adjacent to the Ocean Gateway Terminal. Street parking is available on Commercial Street.

If you're inspired to get on the water, launch a canoe or kayak from Portland's East End Beach or nearby boat launch (where kayaks and canoes are seasonally available for rent). Ample parking is just up the hill from the boat launch on Cutter Street.

NEARBY: Portland's Old Port is a favorite neighborhood with locals and tourists alike. Lobster shacks, restaurants, cafés, ice cream shops, and more can all be found within the waterfront neighborhood.

Trip 4

Fore River Sanctuary and Jewell Falls

Within Portland city limits, this 85-acre nature sanctuary boasts a well-maintained trail network, varied wildlife habitat and Portland's only natural waterfall, the oasis-like Jewell Falls.

Address: 300 Rowe Avenue, Portland
Difficulty: Easy
Distance: 1.0 mile, round-trip
Hours: Dawn to dusk
Fee: Free
Contact: 207-775-2411, trails.org/our-trails/fore-river-sanctuary
Bathrooms: None
Water/Snacks: None
Maps: USGS Portland South quad; trails.org/our-trails/fore-river-sanctuary/
Directions by Car: From I-295, Exit 5B, take Maine 22W/Congress Street west for 0.5 mile. Take a right onto Stevens Avenue, then a left onto Capisic Street in 0.3 mile. Continue 1.3 miles and turn left onto Brighton Avenue. Take the first left onto Rowe Avenue and follow that to the end of the dead-end street and the park's north entrance, where parking is available (43° 39.584′ N, 70° 17.227′ W). If this parking area is full or you want a longer hike through other areas of Fore River Sanctuary than the one described, park at the south entrance at the Maine Orthopedics building at 1601 Congress Street (at the corner of Frost Street), and follow the Congress Street sidewalk to the marked trailhead about 450 feet to the west.

Portlanders introduced to Fore River Sanctuary's Jewell Falls for the first time do a double take. Yes: it's been in your backyard this whole time! While it isn't the largest, most impressive falls in the state, its oasis-like quality makes it the perfect destination when you want a dose of nature without going far from downtown Portland.

From the well-marked trailhead on Rowe Avenue, take the 0.5-mile Jewell Falls Trail, which begins on a slight ridge that runs parallel to train tracks. This narrow, exposed part of the trail cuts through grassland that is a popular habitat for butterflies and common garter snakes. Remember, there are no venomous snakes in Maine, so feel free to stop and say hello. If you find a snake, move

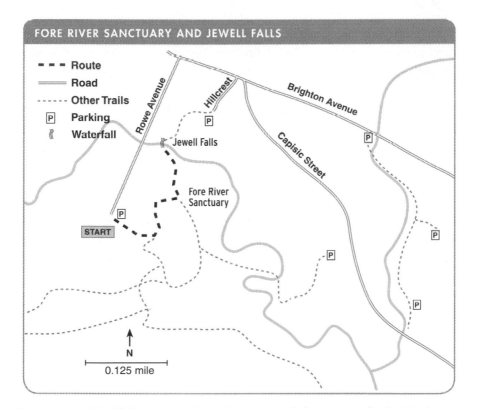

Route
Road
Other Trails
P   Parking
꙰   Waterfall

Rowe Avenue

Hillcrest

Brighton Avenue

Capisic Street

P

P

꙰ Jewell Falls

Fore River
Sanctuary

P

START

P

P

P

P

N

0.125 mile

slowly, watch it carefully, and appreciate the ways it benefits humans by prey-ing on bugs, grubs, rodents, and other pests. Most likely, the snake will quickly slither from the trail once it senses your presence: it's more afraid of you than you could possibly be of it!

At the trail junction in just over 0.1 mile, bear left as the trail dips into the open and beautiful forest, full of maples, evergreens, and ferns. From here, good signage and a wide path over gentle terrain lead all the way to the falls. Kids will light up when they see multiple streams of water cascading down the rocky steps. During springtime or after heavy rains, the water flows more mightily than it does at other times of year; however, the water flows year-round, making this a lovely destination no matter the month.

Get up-close-and-personal with the falls by splashing around in the pools below, or comfortably view it from afar. A stone bench set back from the water pays homage to Tom Jewell, who co-founded Portland Trails and donated this tract of land. To check out Jewell Falls from above, head up the stone staircase that runs parallel to the falls and leads to a wooden bridge spanning the width of the cascade. The trail beyond the bridge continues toward another trailhead at Hillcrest Avenue.

PLAN B: The entire Fore River Sanctuary is open to mountain bikers, on-leash dogs are allowed in some areas, and four separate entrances lead into the Sanctuary from different directions. Though Jewell Falls is a must-see destination, another favorite is the marshland where the river and ocean meet. Kids will love the varied trail, which includes multiple bridges and long boardwalks over towering cattails. During fall, breezes send their fluffy seed heads adrift. Also, stop by the Congress Street trailhead for a history lesson on the Cumberland and Oxford Canal, which opened in 1832, and its role in Maine's shipping before the railroad came to town.

NEARBY: Being so close to downtown Portland, there are myriad options of things to do nearby. Popular with kids are the Children's Museum and Theatre of Maine and the Portland Public Library, which has an excellent children's section with play area.

MORE PORTLAND TRAILS

If you're looking for an easy way to explore another area of Portland Trails' 50-mile network, head over to Capisic Brook Trail from Fore River. Follow a path from Frost Street to Riverview Street, walk the length of Riverview Street to Capisic Street and enter Capisic Brook Trail via the Macy Street entrance. There, you'll find good views of Capisic Pond, Portland's largest freshwater pond. It's a great place to go ice skating in winter and bird-watching year-round. The 0.5-mile trail runs parallel to the lake and has a moderate slope, so it's a good place to venture if your party includes a wheelchair or stroller.

Trip 5

Peaks Island

Take a 20-minute ferry to a paved bike loop around a picturesque island, light spelunking in historic World War II bunkers, and attractive beaches.

Address: 56 Commercial Street, Portland (ferry landing)
Difficulty: Easy
Distance: 4.0 miles, round-trip
Hours: Contact Casco Bay Lines for Peaks Island ferry schedule
Fee: Free for day use; contact Casco Bay Lines for ferry fees
Contact: Portland Trails, 207-775-2411, trails.org/our-trails/peaks-island-loop; Casco Bay Peaks Island Ferry (ferry fees and schedule), 207-774-7871, cascobaylines.com/schedules/peaks-island-schedule; Brad's Bike Rental & Repair (bike rentals on Peaks Island), 207-766-5631
Bathrooms: None
Water/Snacks: None
Maps: USGS Portland East quad; trails.org/our-trails/peaks-island-loop
Directions by Car: From I-295, Exit 7, take US 1A/Franklin Street south for 0.8 miles to the Casco Bay Lines terminal and take the ferry to Peaks Island. Check the schedule online, as it changes seasonally; some launches accommodate cars, others just passengers and bikes. From the Peaks Island ferry landing, walk 0.1 mile to the first intersection with Island Avenue, where the loop trail begins (43° 39.325′ N, 70° 11.870′ W).

Peaks Island was once known as the Coney Island of Maine. Today, it is a small town neighborhood within the city of Portland, a place where kid-run lemonade stands are plentiful in summertime and you can still find flowers or honey for sale at the end of a driveway (on the honor system, of course). Tourists flock here in the warmer months to take in the views of Casco Bay, explore the few quirky museums and galleries, and get a taste for laid-back island living. The ferry—a 20-minute crossing from downtown Portland—runs rain or shine throughout the year, making this an accessible destination anytime you're in the area. Bikes are available for rent on the island near the ferry terminal.

The 4.0-mile bike loop follows a paved road that is mostly flat and waterfront, although it does dip into residential streets in places. The road is shared

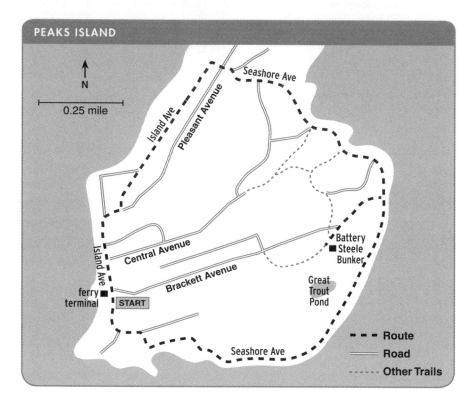

with cars, but there is minimal traffic. From the intersection at Island Avenue, mount your bike and take a right. Continue for 0.2 mile and take your second right onto Whitehead Street. Bike 0.25 mile and take your second right onto Seashore Avenue; follow this street until it ends at the northeastern part of the island.

As you cruise along Seashore Avenue, look for the benches posted at scenic pullouts, offering great resting spots. The sea beyond is a mecca for wildlife and boaters. Keep your eyes pealed for seals, dolphins, and harbor porpoises popping up between Casco Bay's prolific lobster buoys, sailboats, and tankers.

After traveling approximately 1.0 mile along Seashore Avenue, plan to dismount your bicycles and explore the Battery Steele, one of the largest gun batteries ever built in the United States. Though currently preserved as a historic site by the Peaks Island Land Preserve, the World War II battery was once considered critical to protecting Casco Bay. Signage on the west side of Seashore Avenue marks the trailhead. The trail itself is just a few hundred yards, primarily through wet lowlands, over a narrow boardwalk. The battery rises out of the scrubby vegetation like a giant mouth, ready to gobble up anything that dares to enter. This dark, damp place is best explored by older children, armed with flashlights. Those who embrace a little spelunking will love investigating the multiple rooms branching off the primary tunnel. What do they think is behind the heavy, locked doors? ECHO! ECHO...echo!

Back on your bikes, continue on Seashore Avenue to its end and turn left onto Trefethen Avenue. Go 0.1 mile down a steep hill and turn left onto Island Avenue, which leads you back to the ferry terminal. Be sure to check the returning ferry schedule in advance, as ferry times change seasonally.

PLAN B: The ferry runs rain or shine, so don't be afraid to explore the island if the clouds open. When biking isn't in the cards, plan to walk the perimeter loop, or you can always rent a covered golf cart (a popular mode of transportation on Peaks) from Island Tours (207-653-2549).

NEARBY: A few restaurants, gift shops, and galleries are clustered near the Peaks Island ferry terminal. Stroll along Island Avenue to find a gem gallery and the Umbrella Cover Museum. Yes, that's right, this museum is all about sheaths that cover umbrellas! From floral and plaid covers to handmade and international ones, you'll be surprised there is so much to know about umbrella covers!

The state boasts more than a dozen coastal fortifications, some of which are great for families to visit. Lookouts, underground tunnels, and narrow passageways add to the allure. Bring a flashlight and be careful of your footing, wherever you venture. These three are the most family-friendly of the bunch.

Fort Williams

1000 Shore Road, Cape Elizabeth; fortwilliamspark.com; near Trips 1, 3, and 4
Home to Portland Head Light—Maine's oldest lighthouse—Fort Williams Park offers more to explore than only its historic fort. Wide, well-maintained cliff-side trails offer excellent walking opportunities for everyone, including those in strollers and wheelchairs. The park boasts a small beach, tennis courts, a playground, picnic tables, barbecue grills, and a kid-friendly arboretum. During the cold winter months, this is a great destination for sledding, snowshoeing, and cross-country skiing. The two most popular historical highlights are Battery Blair and Erasmus Keys Battery, which is open for exploration May through October.

Fort Popham

10 Perkins Farm Land, Phippsburg, 207-389-1335 (in-season only); near Trips 10 and 11
This semicircular granite fort was originally constructed for use during the Civil War, though it was never finished. Today, it is a well-preserved historic site overlooking a scenic tidal reach. Children will enjoy climbing the many sets of stairs, peering out the windows, and trying to find the hidden chambers. Combine this historic gem with a visit to the popular and nearby Popham Beach State Park and Morse Mountain (Trip 11) for a full day of fun.

Fort Knox

740 Fort Knox Road, Prospect, fortknox.maineguide.com; near Trips 11-18
Fort Knox is the first and largest granite fort built in Maine, constructed to guard the narrows of the Penobscot River. Troops were stationed here during the Civil and Spanish-American wars, though the fort never saw military action. Today, you can explore its many chambers, spiral staircases, and long, narrow alleys. Guided tours are available, as are multiple interpretive signs. Nearby, head to the Penobscot Narrows Bridge observation tower, which rises 420 feet above sea level and provides breathtaking views of the Penobscot River Valley.

Trip 6

Mackworth Island

A short, easy loop trail circles the scenic island, famous for its fairy village where you, too, can create a fairy house from found natural objects.

Address: Mackworth Island, Falmouth
Difficulty: Easy
Distance: 1.25 miles, round-trip
Hours: 6 A.M. to dusk
Fee: $2 adult Maine residents; $3 nonresident adults; $1 children ages 5–12
Contact: Maine Bureau of Public Lands, 207-688-4172, parksandlands.com
Bathrooms: Restrooms near trailhead
Water/Snacks: None
Maps: USGS Portland East quad; trails.org/our-trails/mackworth-island-trail
Directions by Car: From I-295, Exit 9, merge onto US 1N/Veranda Street toward Falmouth Foreside. In 1.2 miles, turn right onto Andrews Avenue; follow Governor Baxter School for the Deaf signs through a residential area and over a causeway before connecting to Mackworth Island. Check in at the guardhouse for a trail brochure and to see if parking is available (43° 41.330′ N, 70° 14.140′ W).

As soon as you set foot on 100-acre Mackworth Island, it's easy to see why the trailhead parking lot is often full. Its close proximity to Portland offers visitors quick and easy access to the splendid natural world. But it's something more than that: from its unique blend of human and natural history to its famous fairy village, this place is magical. Plan to visit on a weekday or during non-peak hours, early in the morning or late in the day, as parking is *very* limited.

The guard at the end of the causeway—who has manned his post for the past ten years and weaves poetry about the island (see "The Fairy Question")—will let you know whether or not parking is available. If not, consider a Plan B or a nearby trip, including Gilsland Farm Audubon Center just a few miles away (Trip 7) or Portland's Eastern Promenade (Trip 3).

The 1.25-mile round-trip trail encircling the island has a prominently marked trailhead on the south end of the parking lot, near the restrooms and fee deposit box. In this open area, native wildflowers are seasonally abundant, including wood anemones, baneberry, goldenrod, and nightshade. The wide,

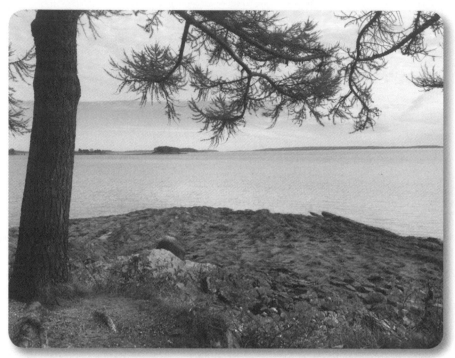

Catch views of Casco Bay around every corner of the Mackworth Island trail.

level trail has a surface of compacted soil. Aside from the occasional rock or root, nothing about the trail impedes stroller or wheelchair accessibility.

As the trail moves into the forest edge, begin to look for signs of wildlife. The oak and pine forest here provides food and shelter for grouse, foxes, rabbits, skunks, squirrels, sparrows, warblers, and many more species. The trail offers plenty of places to rest and listen quietly to nature's sounds: there are multiple benches and a few large swings with sweeping views of Casco Bay.

Three separate sets of stairs at different locations along the island trail lead to the rocky beach. Here, the intertidal zone offers much for little fingers to explore. Can kids carefully lift rockweed and stone to find green crabs hiding below? In the tide pools, can they find periwinkles, barnacles, and blue mussels? Do they recognize any of the shorebirds, including great blue herons, eider ducks, and cormorants?

Back on the trail, at the north end of the island, a short side trail leads to one of the island's unique features, the pet cemetery. Here, former Maine Governor Percival Baxter (who donated Mackworth Island to the state of Maine in 1946) buried his beloved Irish setters and his horse.

Another unusual feature of Mackworth is the Fairy House Village, located just beyond the pet cemetery on the trail's inland side, marked with a sign stating that it "provides fairies with cottages during their visit to the island." Take time to admire the builders' creativity and, if inspired to do so, create fairy houses of your own. If you do choose to add to the village, use only fallen items already on the ground, such as twigs, acorns, pinecones, and pebbles. As we all know, fairies look down upon hurting any living thing, including trees and shrubs.

Continue along the trail as it curves southwest back toward the parking area. Reference your trail brochure often to learn about the island's other unique features, including the hollow but mighty Listening Tree, which has a growth inside resembling a giant ear.

PLAN B: Within the greater Portland area, there are myriad alternatives for getting your family outdoors, including paddling Scarborough Marsh (Trip 1), biking Portland's Back Cove and Eastern Promenade Trails (Trip 3) or hiking at Gilsland Farm Audubon Center (Trip 7) or Fore River Sanctuary (Trip 4).

NEARBY: Head north on Route 1 to find multiple dining options and grocery stores.

"THE FAIRY QUESTION"

by Mackworth Island Gatekeeper Steve King

> *You ask if there are Fairies here.*
> *Well, I can tell you Yes my Dear.*
> *Cause here are friends that help them be.*
> *Like tallest pines and sparkling sea.*
> *Like fox and hare and doe and fawn*
> *And ducks that dive*
> *And sun at dawn.*
> *Like bay so bright*
> *And starry night.*
> *So yes my Dear*
> *There's Fairies here.*

Trip 7

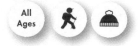

Gilsland Farm Audubon Center

Five minutes from downtown Portland, this year-round sanctuary offers a variety of habitats, gentle trails, and an indoor nature center.

Address: 20 Gilsland Farm Road, Falmouth
Difficulty: Easy
Distance: 0.7–2.5 miles, round-trip
Hours: Dawn to dusk; Audubon Center open Monday–Saturday, 9 A.M.–5 P.M.
and Sundays and holidays, noon to 4 P.M.
Fee: Free
Contact: 207-781-2330, maineaudubon.org/our-locations/gilsland-farm
Bathrooms: At the Audubon Center
Water/Snacks: Water fountain at the Audubon Center (no snacks)
Maps: USGS Cumberland County quad; mainetrailfinder.com/trails/gilsland-farm
Directions by Car: From I-295, Exit 9, continue 1.9 miles north on US 1 and turn left onto Gilsland Farm Road at the Audubon sign, immediately before the intersection of US 1 and US 88. Gilsland Farm Road leads to a parking lot with ample spaces. Access the trailhead across from the Gilsland Farm Audubon Center (43° 42.362′ N, 70° 14.432′ W).

Year-round exploration is easy at Gilsland Farm, home to Maine Audubon's headquarters, located just a few minutes from downtown Portland. Upon arrival, it's hard to choose where to start: both the modern Audubon Center and the trails beckon, and both are worth a visit. Begin your journey at the center, open seven days a week, to learn more about the property, its history and trails, and the nature-related exhibits on display. Kids will likely beeline for the Children's Discovery Room, where they can observe live turtles, play with eco-themed puzzles and games, and try their eyes at bird-watching through kid-friendly binoculars out the huge windows facing multiple bird-feeding stations. Adjacent to this room are the reading library and conference room, which contain a large collection of mounted specimens of Maine birds and mammals, including several extinct species. If children venture into this area, make sure an adult is supervising.

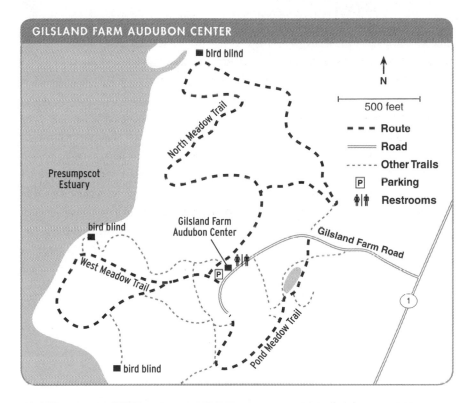

bird blind

N

500 feet

- - - Route
=== Road
----- Other Trails
P Parking
Restrooms

North Meadow Trail

Presumpscot
Estuary

bird blind

Gilsland Farm
Audubon Center

Gilsland Farm Road

West Meadow Trail

Pond Meadow Trail

1

bird blind

The well-established trail network begins close to the environmental center, and a large wooden map illustrates the 65-acre sanctuary and its three primary trails—North Meadow Trail, West Meadow Trail, and Pond Meadow Trail. The paths are connected by spur trails and junctions, so it's feasible to trek the complete 2.5-mile network in an afternoon. Doing so will allow you to explore the greatest diversity of habitat, ranging from woodlands and meadow to pond and shoreline. The trails stay open year-round, and snowshoes are available for rent at the environmental center.

Take 0.6-mile Pond Meadow Trail as it winds behind the Audubon Center through mature stands of red oak and hemlock dating back more than a century, enter into younger woods of white ash, red maple, white birch, and trembling aspen, and explore the pond where you may catch glimpse of muskrats and wetland birds. From here, take a spur to 1.2-mile North Meadow Trail, which loops around a meadow that was once used as farmland. To continue the loop, take a spur to the Audubon Center, then link with 0.7-mile West Meadow Trail, which is a great hike on its own if you have time for only one. It meanders through a small, forested wetland. Kids will enjoy walking the boardwalks before the trail becomes grassy and enters a field. Follow the trail up to the bluffs, which overlook the Presumpscot River estuary with views to the Portland skyline beyond. A few simple benches provide good resting and snack spots. As with the other trails in the network, natural history signage dots the landscape here, helping hikers identify native trees and shrubs.

Eventually West Meadow Trail joins with spur trails, each of which leads to an observation blind for spotting waterfowl. In summer, look for flocks of migrant shorebirds gathering on the mudflats, especially when a low tide exposes a plethora of marine life. Even if your little ones lack the attention span to observe birds, they'll enjoy the fort-like feeling inspired by the observation blind. The blind offers a good vantage point to look back in history: help kids imagine what they would have seen during the thousands of years that this land was home to the Wabanakis and their ancestors. Can they envision the native peoples stooped over the estuary's vast tidal flats, harvesting shellfish or fishing for mackerel and striped bass? Where do they imagine the first peoples took shelter during the dead of winter? To conclude your hike, continue on West Meadow Trail, which loops back toward the parking area.

PLAN B: There is plenty to do right at Gilsland Farm if hiking doesn't appeal to your party. You can shop for books, toys, and Maine-made gifts at the Maine Audubon Nature Store within the environmental center, or have a picnic lunch in the butterfly garden nearby. Farther afield, Mackworth Island (Trip 6) is less than 2 miles away and offers an excellent option for exploring different habitats, including beaches.

NEARBY: Head north on US 1 for 1 mile to the town of Falmouth or south on US 1 for 4 miles to Portland. Both have numerous restaurants, shops, and other amenities.

Trip 8

Bradbury Mountain

Without much effort, catch great views at this popular, easy-to-access destination, the perfect place for introducing kids to hiking.

Address: 528 Hallowell Road, Pownal
Difficulty: Easy–Moderate
Distance: 1.3 miles, round-trip
Hours: 9 A.M. to sunset
Fee: $3 adult Maine residents, $4.50 adult nonresidents, $1 children ages 5–11
Contact: 207-688-4712, bradburymountain.com
Bathrooms: Near the parking lots
Water/Snacks: None
Maps: USGS North Pownal quad; bradburymountain.com/trail-maps.html
Directions by Car: From I-295, take Exit 22 toward ME 125/ME 136 N/Mallet Drive and follow signs to Bradbury. In 0.2 mile, turn left onto Durham Road. Follow this road (which becomes Pownal Road, then Elmwood Road) for 4.4 miles to the blinking light at the intersection of ME 9 and Elmwood Road. Turn right onto ME 9. In 0.5 mile, arrive at Bradbury State Park, where there is ample parking (43° 45.942′ N, 70° 17.854′ W).

If you're looking for a mountain that even the littlest legs can climb, Bradbury Mountain is the place to start. Located just a few miles off of the highway near Freeport, this 800-acre state park is easy to access and full of amenities, including an extensive playground, a picnic area, and bathrooms at the mountain's base near the large parking lot. You also don't have to go far to get great views, which makes this mountain a must-do for families exploring Maine.

For the shortest, most direct route to the top, take 0.3-mile Summit Trail, which is well marked and easily accessible from the picnic area near the main parking lot. This hiking-only trail winds up through shady forest, over some rock staircases and bare roots. Though moderately steep, the route is easily navigable by the whole family, including little explorers, particularly when they realize how close they are to the mountaintop! Leaving the forest, the trail reaches the wide, flat, bald rock summit, where there is ample space to spread out a packed picnic and enjoy the scenery, even on the busiest of weekends.

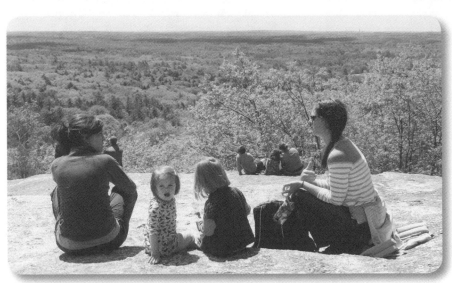

From the wide, bald rock summit of Bradbury Mountain, the forest seems to extend forever.

On a clear day the view stretches as far as Casco Bay, and the fall foliage from this vantage point is not to be missed. During autumn months, look for migrating eagles riding the thermals. Spring is the best time to catch a glimpse of migrating hawks: from mid-March through mid-May, birders descend on the summit to take daily raptor counts, particularly of Northern Goshawks.

Multiple trails descend the mountain. For a more gradual slope than that of the Summit Trail, take 1.0-mile Northern Loop Trail, which is flat and wide enough to accommodate a robust stroller. This is a multiuse trail, popular with mountain bikers, hikers with dogs, and even horseback riders. And keep your eyes out for an old cattle pound that still stands nearby: early settlers used the stone walls to hold in cattle, sheep, and pigs.

Remember, there are plenty of trails to choose from when exploring this large state park. Those on the west side of the mountain, accessible from the main parking lot, are more appropriate for hikers and families, while routes on the eastern slope are popular with mountain bikers.

PLAN B: When rain strikes or the bugs are just too much for your tyke, consider heading to Wolfe's Neck Farm (Trip 9, Plan B), another destination near Freeport. Here, you can take cover inside barns and get to know the farm animals while you wait to venture outside

NEARBY: If amenities are needed, head into downtown Freeport. There, kids can get inside the fish tank observation bubble at the L.L. Bean flagship store or even tour the ever popular Wilbur's Chocolate Factory.

Trip 9

Wolfe's Neck Woods State Park

This coastal treasure offers 5 miles of easy forest and shore-side walking trails, including a wheelchair- and stroller-accessible path. Bring your binoculars!

Address: 426 Wolfe's Neck Road, Freeport
Difficulty: Easy
Distance: 2.1 miles, round-trip
Hours: 9 A.M. to sunset, Memorial Day to Labor Day
Fee: $3 adult Maine residents, $4.50 adult nonresidents, $1 children ages 5–11
Contact: 207-865-4465, parksandlands.com
Bathrooms: Restrooms at trailhead
Water/Snacks: None
Maps: USGS Freeport quad; parksandlands.com
Directions by Car: From I-295 N, Exit 20, follow signs for Freeport. Travel 1.3 miles north on US 1 and turn right on Bow Street (across from L.L. Bean's flagship store). In 2.4 miles, turn right onto Wolfe's Neck Road. Continue for 2.0 miles, following signs for the state park. Turn left at the park entrance and continue toward the large parking area (43° 49.359′ N, 70° 5.065′ W).

Drive five minutes away from Freeport's bustling shopping district, and Wolfe's Neck Woods State Park transports you into the tranquil natural world. This 245-acre park has 5 miles of easy walking trails, clean and modern restrooms, a picnic area, and diverse ecosystems, including mature hemlock and white pine forests, a salt marsh estuary, and the rocky shorelines of the Harraseeket River and Casco Bay. Named after the land's early European settlers, Henry and Rachel Wolfe and established in 1972, this park is now considered one of Maine's coastal treasures.

Explore the best of the trail system by setting off on Casco Bay Trail. From the north end of the parking area, enter the woods to the right of the big wooden sign. This popular trail offers an easy, short walk to the ocean.

To extend the trip and explore majestic stands of mature forest, add on the 1.8-mile Harraseeket loop. Just a few hundred feet after entering the forest, Casco Bay Trail meets Harraseeket Trail. Bear right here, ducking farther into the woods. Cross Old Woods Road Trail, Power Line Trail, and Wolfe's

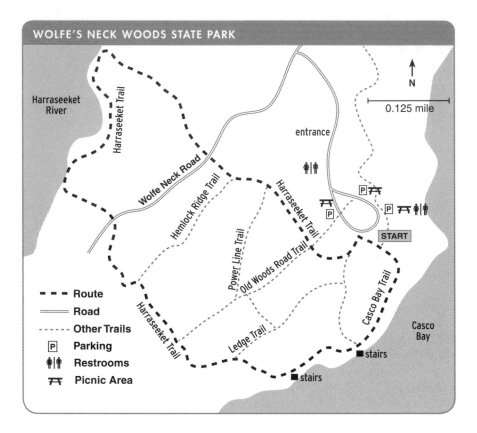

Harraseeket
River

Harraseeket Trail

Wolfe Neck Road

Hemlock Ridge Trail

Harraseeket Trail

entrance

0.125 mile

N

START

Power Line Trail

Old Woods Road Trail

Casco Bay Trail

Casco
Bay

- - - Route

=== Road

----- Other Trails

P Parking

Restrooms

Picnic Area

Harraseeket Trail

Ledge Trail

stairs

stairs

Neck Road. (Note that Wolfe's Neck Road is the road you traveled by car to access the park, so beware of vehicles when crossing.) After a gradual descent through lovely mature forest, the trail traverses the cliffs above the Harraseeket River, offering views of South Freeport and its marina and resident boats. Here, rocky ledges make for great rest spots, but take care that kids don't get too close to the edge. Leaving the shoreline, the trail ducks back into the forest, over a wooden bridge, and gently uphill before recrossing Wolfe's Neck Road. Bear right at each of the next three trail junctions to stay on Harraseeket Trail and eventually rejoin Casco Bay Trail at the ocean's edge.

At the trail junction of Harraseeket and Casco Bay trails, an interpretive sign points out the animals of the bay, and a set of stairs leads down to the rocky shore. Kids will enjoy exploring the beach here, so plan to stop a while and take in the views of Casco Bay and Cousins, Eagle, and Googins islands. Googins is home to majestic ospreys, who mate for life and summer on the island before making the long flight each fall to South America. To learn more about ospreys and other wildlife who call this area home, consider joining one of the park's many free, naturalist-led programs offered throughout summer and fall. Continue along Casco Bay Trail to return to the trailhead and parking area.

For those visitors exploring the park via wheelchair or stroller, head to the accessible White Pines Trail. Clear signage from the parking lot marks the way.

PLAN B: The 626-acre Wolfe's Neck Farm is a nonprofit saltwater farm open free to the public every day from dawn to dusk. Here, kids can visit the farm animals, learn about agriculture, hike, bike, kayak, canoe, and participate in myriad education and community events. Family drop-in programs are popular on summer Saturdays, including the Family Barnyard program and the Farmer for the Morning program, offering kids the opportunity to learn about, feed, and water the animals. Check the website calendar often for seasonal events, such as the Fall Festival and summertime Maine Lobster Bakes. Bicycles, kayaks, and canoes are available for rent, as are campsites at the family-friendly oceanfront campground. For more information, visit wolfesneckfarm.org or call 207-865-4469.

NEARBY: Downtown Freeport is home to the flagship L.L. Bean store, as well as multiple outlet stores, restaurants, and ice cream shops.

Trip 10

All Ages $ 🚶 🚴 🛶 🏊 ⛺

Hermit Island

Hermit Island offers unparalleled saltwater camping with plentiful sandy beaches, paddling opportunities, hiking trails, and bike-friendly dirt roads—something for the whole family!

Address: Head Beach Road (between Archies Drive and Hermit Island Road), Phippsburg
Difficulty: Easy–Moderate
Distance: Varies
Hours: Open seasonally, May 15–Columbus Day
Fee: Campsite fees vary; reservations required during high season; no day use
Contact: Hermit Island Campground Office, 207-443-2101, hermitisland.com
Bathrooms: Located throughout campground
Water/Snacks: Potable water available at spigots throughout campground; the store at the campground entrance offers an assortment of food and drink
Maps: USGS Small Point quad; hermitisland.com/map.html
Directions by Car: From I-295, Exit 28, take US 1 north for 10.6 miles to the ME 209/ME 216 exit toward Phippsburg. Follow ME 209/ME 216 for 14.5 miles to Hermit Island. Stop at the entrance gate to check in and receive an island map (43° 43.202′ N, 69° 51.114′ W).

Maine's best saltwater camping may be on Hermit Island, a 225-acre peninsula jutting into Casco Bay. Stay at one of 275 family-friendly, seasonal campsites located near sandy beaches, in the forested interior, on rocky cliffs, or along the tidal harbor, each within walking or biking distance of one of six beaches.

Easy to moderate hiking trails lead to the island's most pristine, remote beaches. Wild berries, including gooseberries, blueberries, raspberries, and blackberries, all make great additions to the dinner menu in season! Rig up a fishing pole for the striper and bluefish that can be plentiful in these waters. And be sure the little tykes bring their buckets! Tidepools teem with everything from hermit crabs and snails to sea stars and urchins, and freshwater Lily Pond located in the southern part of the island is a great spot to catch toads and salamanders. Here, be on the lookout for muskrats scrounging for food and beavers building dams.

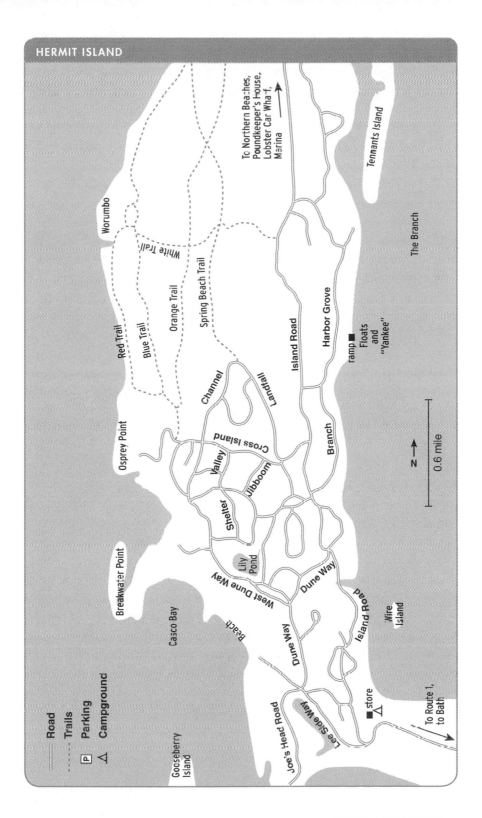

Road
Trails
P Parking
△ Campground

Gooseberry Island

Joe's Head Road

Lee Side Way

■ store
△

To Route 1,
to Bath

Casco Bay

Breakwater Point

Beach

Dune Way

West Dune Way

Dune Way

Island Road

Wire Island

Lily Pond

Shelter

Valley

Jibboom

Cross Island

Branch

N
0.6 mile

Osprey Point

Channel

Landfall

Island Road

Harbor Grove

■ ramp
Floats
and
"Yankee"

Red Trail

Blue Trail

Orange Trail

Spring Beach Trail

White Trail

Worumbo

To Northern Beaches,
Poundkeeper's House,
Lobster Car Wharf,
Marina

Tennants Island

The Branch

Hermit Island's many amenities add to this destination's allure. Warm showers and potable water, located throughout the campground, are included in your campsite fee. The campground's store sells everything from firewood to fresh lobster. The Kelp Shed, across from the store, has an indoor game area and outdoor ping-pong tables and volleyball net. Canoes and rowboats are available for rent. Campsites fill quickly at high season. Make reservations far in advance.

PLAN B: Popham Beach State Park offers a great day trip for campers looking for adventure off the island. The park's long sandy beach draws many a sun-bather and seaside stroller. Consider a low-tide walk to Fox Island, but be sure to consult a tide chart so you don't end up marooned; contact Popham Beach State Park at 207-389-9125 for more information. While in the area, consider venturing 2.0 miles north to Fort Popham State Historic Site, a semicircular granite fort at the mouth of the Kennebec River. Head to nearby Morse Mountain (Trip 11) for a hike and a day at the beach.

NEARBY: The small city of Bath, 15 miles north of Hermit Island, is home to restaurants, shops, boutiques, and galleries, many of which reside on the pedestrian-friendly Front and Centre streets. You might also want to stop by Bath's Maine Maritime Museum, which offers multiple interactive exhibits for kids. For more information, visit mainemaritimemuseum.org.

ABOUT BEAVERS

Most kids will know that the ingenious beavers use trees to build their lodges, dams, sluiceways, and channels; capture water in low-lying areas; and make new ponds. But they also eat the trees! Beavers are vegetarians, so they exist solely on branches, leaves, lily pads, and other aquatic vegetation. Any trees that they don't use for construction in summer get stockpiled at the bottom of the lake for eating later in winter. After the lake freezes over, they swim out of their lodges through passageways beneath the ice, and dive deep to fetch the perfectly preserved branches and leaves at the bottom of the lake. Beavers seal up most of their lodge with mud and leaves so that the wind doesn't make its way through the sticks, but they leave a small hole at the top for ventilation, so on an especially cold day in winter, you just might see a bit of vapor rising out of the top of the lodge—that is the body heat and breath of the beavers!

Trip 11

Morse Mountain

Don't choose between a scenic hike through the woods and a day at the beach; here, you can have it all!

Address: Morse Mountain Road (between ME 216 and Gatehouse Lane), Phippsburg
Difficulty: Easy–Moderate
Distance: 4.0 miles, round-trip
Hours: Dawn to dusk
Fee: Free
Contact: Bates-Morse Conservation Area, 207-786-6078, morseriver.com/MRA_ Bates_Morse_Mountain_Welcome_Bulletin.pdf; The Nature Conservancy Maine, 507-729-5181, nature.org/maine
Bathrooms: None
Water/Snacks: None
Maps: USGS Small Point quad; *Maine Atlas and Gazetteer,* Map 6: E5 (DeLorme)
Directions by Car: From the intersection of US 1 and ME 209 in Bath, travel south on ME 209 toward Phippsburg for 11.2 miles. Continue straight onto ME 216/Small Point Road (driving past the Popham Beach turnoff). After 0.8 mile on ME 216, take a left onto Morse Mountain Road. The small dirt parking lot is located on the left, and trail maps are available at the information kiosk (43° 44.724′ N, 69° 50.230′ W).

This "mountain's" elevation tops out at 180 feet, but the views from here are actually quite impressive, and this destination has more allure than just its summit: the pleasant, gentle hike leads through lovely terrain before opening onto one of Maine's most pristine, spectacular beaches. The variety of terrain and lack of facilities will require you to plan ahead, but the preparation will be well worth the effort.

From the parking area, follow the well-marked, wide old fire road, which is mostly paved with some areas of hard-packed gravel; this section is sturdy-stroller friendly. It leads first through hardwood forest and then passes through wetlands and along the Sprague River Salt Marsh, which provides critical habitat for a wide variety of wildlife. Keep your eyes out for migrating birds, particularly in September and October! At approximately 1.0 mile, the trail

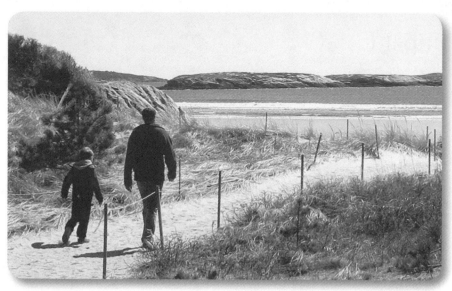
Cross sand dunes at the terminus of Morse Mountain Trail to reach stunning Seawall Beach.

reaches a junction near the summit. To reach the scenic outlook, veer right uphill, following the sign for the viewpoint. The coastline spreads below, as do miles of Maine woods and the winding Sprague River entering the Atlantic Ocean.

After taking in the views, continue back to the trail as it dips down toward Seawall Beach. When the trail opens to the sand dunes, you'll feel as if you've stumbled onto paradise: the white sand beach seems to stretch forever, dotted here and there with driftwood forts. Clear ocean water beckons, so be sure to pack a suit and towel for a quick dip. Enjoy the wild, unspoiled character of this landscape before retracing your steps to the parking lot.

PLAN B: For a spectacular though much more crowded beach, head 5 miles east to Popham Beach State Park. At low tide, consider a walk to Fox Island, but be sure to consult a tide chart so you don't end up marooned; for up-to-date information contact Popham Beach State Park at 207-389-9125.

Other nearby destinations include Hermit Island (Trip 10) and Fort Popham State Historic Site, a semicircular granite fort at the mouth of the Kennebec River.

NEARBY: Thirteen miles north of Morse Mountain is the small city of Bath, where you can find restaurants and shops, as well as the Maine Maritime Museum, which offers multiple interactive exhibits for kids. For more information, visit mainemaritimemuseum.org.

Trip 12

Mount Battie

This fantastic hike offers spectacular views of Camden Harbor and Penobscot Bay, a stone tower, and multiple interpretive signs pointing out the area's historical significance.

Address: Megunticook Street Extension, Camden
Difficulty: Moderate
Distance: 1.0 mile, round-trip
Hours: 9 A.M. to sunset
Fee: $3 adult Maine residents, $4.50 adult nonresidents, $1 children ages 5–11
Contact: Camden Hills State Park, 207-236-3109, parksandlands.com
Bathrooms: None
Water/Snacks: None
Maps: USGS Camden quad; *Maine Mountains Trail Map*, Map 4: C1 (AMC); maine.gov/dacf/parks/docs/fpl/camdentrails.pdf
Directions by Car: From the junction of US 1 and ME 52 in Camden, drive north on ME 52 for approximately 100 yards, then turn right onto Megunticook Street (a residential road). Drive to the end of the road, where trailhead parking is available at the gravel turnout on the left (44° 12.974′ N, 69° 4.170′ W).

Mount Battie offers one of the most stunning views of the craggy Maine coastline. It's no wonder that the 0.5-mile trail to the summit has long been a favorite with families, particularly considering the castle-like stone tower that beckons at the top and the views of Camden and Penobscot Bay along the way.

From the northern side of the parking area, blue-blazed Mount Battie Trail heads into forested terrain. The ascent is gentle at first before quickly becoming more challenging as the trail switches back and forth uphill. Ledge outcrops offer natural stepping stones. In 0.2 mile, the trail opens to its first view of the surrounding Camden hills and a large ledge stone offers the perfect resting spot before continuing on the climb. Terrain becomes steeper after this; children may need to use all fours in order to scale the short set of 15-foot cliffs. Beyond the cliffs, the trail emerges from the forest and opens onto more barren, rocky ledges. From here upward, the views get better and better (as do the blueberries, in season). Take time to enjoy them in relative solitude:

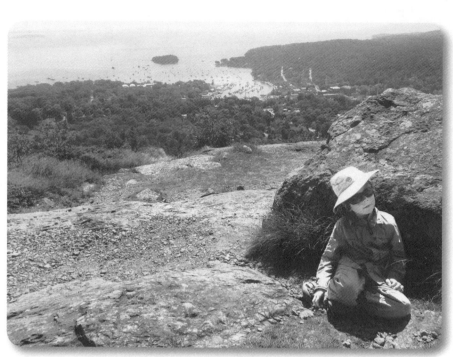

Exposure increases as you approach Mount Battie's summit, but there are still plenty of places to seek shelter and take a break from the climb. (Photo courtesy Jeanne Short)

soon, you'll be sharing the panorama with the throngs of people who access the summit by car.

Reach the 800-foot summit just 0.5 mile from the trailhead. Multiple interpretive signs orient you to the landscape, highlighting the various islands that rise from the water below. On a clear day, this 360-degree panorama rivals any in the state.

The impressive stone tower perched on top of the summit was erected in 1921 as a World War I memorial. The tower's foundation utilizes rock from a grand hotel that stood in this exact spot before being damaged by fire in 1918. Can you imagine looking out your hotel window and seeing this view? Scale the tower via a spiral staircase within. Small children will need extra supervision here, as the ascent is steep and the railing was not built to today's standards. To return to the trailhead, retrace your steps back down the mountain.

PLAN B: If hiking isn't in your cards but you still want to take in the spectacular views of the summit, you can drive to the top (just don't tell the kids this if you *do* plan to hike). From Camden Center, head north on US 1 for approximately 1 mile to Camden Hills State Park on your left. Check in and pay the entrance fee at the gatehouse before proceeding up the paved Mount Battie Auto Road to the parking area at the summit.

Other popular hiking trips nearby include Mount Megunticook, Maiden Cliff Trail, and Nature Trail. For more information, contact the state park.

Consider taking a ferry or water taxi to the local islands of Penobscot Bay, including Vinalhaven, North Haven, Islesboro, and Matinicus. Visiting any of these islands will give you a true sense of what it is like to live in a traditional New England seafaring community.

NEARBY: Camden is a quintessential Maine coastal town and summer tourist destination, with many attractive dining options, galleries, and museums (including the largest lighthouse museum in the nation). In nearby Rockland, children will delight in the Coastal Children's Museum.

INSPIRING A POET

As legend has it, the celebrated American poet Edna St. Vincent Millay (1892-1950) wrote the famous poem "Renascence" while enjoying the view from the summit of Mount Battie. The opening lines of the poem (below) are engraved in a bronze plaque set in stone at the top of the mountain.

"RENASCENCE"

All I could see from where I stood
Was three long mountains and a wood;
I turned and looked another way,
And saw three islands in a bay.
So with my eyes I traced the line
Of the horizon, thin and fine,
Straight around till I was come
Back to where I'd started from;
And all I saw from where I stood
Was three long mountains and a wood.

Trip 13

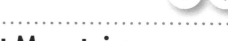

Ages 8+

Penobscot Mountain

From boardwalks and bridges to stone staircases and sheer cliff faces, this varied terrain will keep older children engaged as they seek the scenic summit.

Address: Park Loop Road, Seal Harbor
Difficulty: Challenging
Distance: 3.2 miles, round-trip
Hours: No posted hours; contact park for seasonal road and trail closures
Fee: $20 per vehicle; $5 per adult without a vehicle, including bicyclists and pedestrians (children under 15 are free)
Contact: Acadia National Park, 207-288-3338, nps.gov/acad
Bathrooms: Restrooms at Jordan Pond House
Water/Snacks: Restaurant and gift shop at Jordan Pond House
Maps: USGS Southwest Harbor quad; *Acadia National Park Discovery Map* (AMC), Eastern Mount Desert Island: E5–E6
Directions by Car: From Bar Harbor, take ME 233 to the Cadillac Mountain entrance of Acadia National Park. Follow the signs for Cadillac Mountain and then the sign for Jordan Pond (7.0 miles) (44° 19.158′ N, 68° 15.435′ W).

Few of Acadia National Park's visitors venture up Penobscot Mountain—a hike offering some of Acadia's most interesting terrain and sweeping panoramic views. While sections of the hike will challenge even experienced youngsters, the rewards and the grand sense of accomplishment are well worth the effort.

The trail begins near the historic Jordan Pond House. Facing the house, walk behind the left side of the building to the trailhead marker. Follow the trail into the woods, almost immediately crossing the carriage trail. Take care when crossing, as this is a popular route for bicyclists (see Trip 15). The trail then crosses Jordan Stream via a small footbridge.

From this crossing onward, you leave the hustle and bustle of Jordan Pond House behind as you forge farther into the woods and up the mountain. Much of the terrain for the first 0.25 mile is comprised of stone stairs. At 0.5 mile, the trail reaches an intersection with Jordan Cliffs Trail. Here, continue to the left, up Penobscot Mountain Trail to another intersection with the carriage trail.

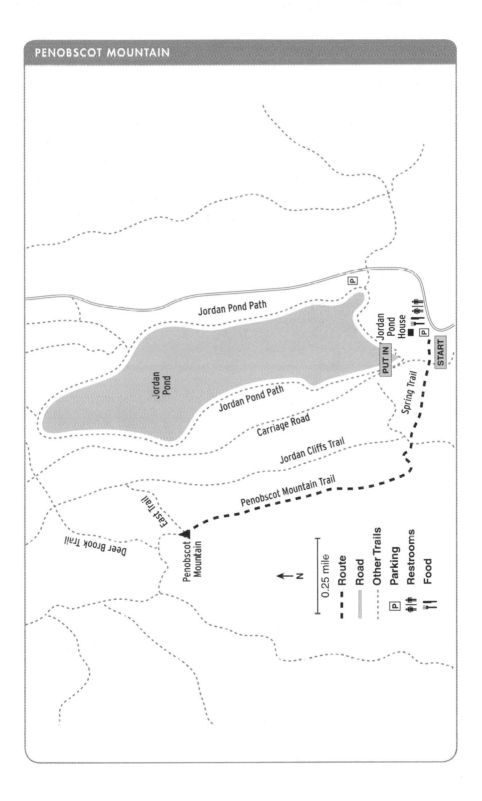

Jordan Pond Path

Jordan Pond

Jordan Pond Path

Carriage Road

Jordan Cliffs Trail

Penobscot Mountain Trail

Jordan Pond House

PUT IN

Spring Trail

START

East Trail

Deer Brook Trail

Penobscot Mountain

0.25 mile

← N

- - - Route
———— Road
· · · · · Other Trails
Ⓟ Parking
🚹 Restrooms
🍴 Food

(Again, take caution when crossing.) The trail picks up on the other side, via a trail marker that reads Spring Trail.

The Spring Trail section is the climb's most interesting and most challenging. It begins as another set of stone stairs, then follows a narrow stone ledge flanked with a sheer rock face on one side and a drop-off on the other. There is a wooden guardrail protecting you from the drop-off, but children should proceed with extra caution and supervision. After crossing a wooden bridge, the rocky ledge continues briefly before bringing you to another interesting feature and the most difficult section of the hike by far—a slot between large boulders requiring a hand-over-hand scramble. Take your time and watch your footing as you squeeze your way through the rocks and up this short, steep section.

The trail soon opens to an impressive viewpoint with a stone makeshift bench and a stunning view—the perfect place to rest and refuel for the second half of the ascent. From here, the view of Jordan Pond is a sight to behold. Can children imagine the native Penobscot people, for whom the mountain is named, traveling across the pond in their birch-bark canoes? The Penobscots are one of two native peoples who lived in the Acadia region before European settlement.

After soaking in the views, continue climbing up the trail, which quickly rises above treeline. Follow cairns and blue blazes to stay on track as you travel up the open mountain face. The views get more and more spectacular as you climb: the mountain's summit looms above; below, the Atlantic Ocean and its islands spread as far as the eye can see. After tagging the summit marker, 1.6 miles from the trailhead, take a few photos and revel in the sense of accomplishment that comes with finishing a challenging hike, then retrace your steps back down the mountain.

PLAN B: An alternate and much easier hike from this trailhead is Shore Trail, which circumnavigates the pond, following the water's edge in a 3.3-mile loop. Signage near the parking area directs you to the trail. Jordan Pond itself has some of the most exceptionally clear water recorded in Maine. While swimming is not allowed, nonmotorized boats are. Launch a canoe or kayak via the Jordan Pond North parking lot, a short distance from the trailhead parking.

NEARBY: The historical and picturesque Jordan Pond House restaurant, overlooking Jordan Pond, has been serving the public since the 1870s and is the only full-service restaurant within Acadia National Park. The restaurant has a full menu, as well as stunning views of Penobscot Mountain and the Bubbles.

Trip 14

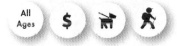

The Bubbles

Kids will delight in the huge, precariously perched boulder and the surrounding panoramas of the Gulf of Maine and Jordan Pond.

Address: Park Loop Road, Bar Harbor
Difficulty: Easy–Moderate
Distance: 1.0 mile, round-trip
Hours: No posted hours; contact park for seasonal road and trail closures
Fee: $20 per vehicle; $5 per adult without a vehicle, including bicyclists and pedestrians (children under 15 are free)
Contact: Acadia National Park, 207-288-3338, nps.gov/acad; Island Explorer Bike Express, 207-667-5796, exploreacadia.com/bikeexpress.htm
Bathrooms: None
Water/Snacks: None
Maps: USGS Southwest Harbor quad; *Acadia National Park Discovery Map* (AMC), Eastern Mount Desert Island: D6, E6
Directions by Car: From ME 3 and the Acadia National Park Visitor Center in Hulls Cove, head south on the Park Loop Road for 6.0 miles to the Bubble Rock parking lot (44° 20.465′ N, 68° 14.981′ W), 1.0 mile beyond the parking area for Bubble Pond.

Rising above the north end of Jordan Pond, North Bubble and South Bubble look just the way they sound—two perfect bubbles of pink granite symmetrically rising from the earth. While more experienced hikers prepared for a longer hike can easily summit both in a day (see Plan B), start with the South Bubble. It is slightly smaller and more accessible, with arguably greater views and features at the summit.

From the well-marked trailhead at the western side of the parking lot, trails for both North and South Bubble begin together, gradually ascending through deciduous forest on a well-worn path. The compacted dirt terrain soon gives way to a natural staircase of terraced log and stone. Ample signage directs you toward the Bubbles as you continue on your climb. Just after the 0.3-mile mark, North and South Bubble trails diverge: stay left (southeast) toward South Bubble. As the trail rises above tree level, follow infrequent blue blazes on rocks to keep your bearing.

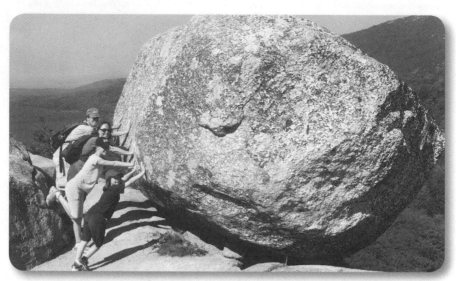

The South Bubble's large glacial erratic left over from the last ice age is not as easy to push off the steep cliff face as it looks...but you're welcome to try!

Reach the 768-foot baldface summit (0.5 mile). The true kid-magnet, Bubble Rock (sometimes called Balance Rock), lies slightly below the summit, as do the views of Jordan Pond, Eagle Lake, Penobscot and Cadillac mountains, and even the Atlantic Ocean. Descend eastward on a marked spur trail to reach this glacial erratic within a few hundred feet. The precariously perched boulder looks as though it could easily roll off the mountain at any moment. (Don't worry, it won't! It weighs 14 tons.) While admirers are welcome to get up close and personal with the rock—which is estimated to have been deposited here by a glacier approximately 10,000 years ago—children should explore the ledges surrounding it with caution and supervision. Return to the summit and then retrace your steps back toward the trailhead and parking area (1.0 mile).

PLAN B: When in Bubble territory, why not explore both? Descend from the South Bubble summit via Bubbles Divide Trail. Instead of continuing straight down toward the parking area, take a left (heading north) at the trail junction for North Bubble Trail. Reach the summit in just over 0.1 mile. This adds 0.2 mile to the route above.

NEARBY: The town of Bar Harbor, 7 miles from the Bubble Rock parking lot, is a lively tourist destination, offering plenty for families to do, see, eat, and enjoy. Those interested in marine life can venture to the marina at the end of Main Street and sign up for tours to see everything from puffins and seals to island lighthouses.

The best way to learn the interconnectedness of all living things is to see first-hand how organisms interact with their environments. When planning trips, try to find information about where you are going—what habitats you'll be exploring and what plants and animals you might expect to see. Kids will be more excited about the adventure ahead when they have particular plants and animals to look for. The very best tools kids have for learning about ecology are their senses—which don't add weight to the backpack. Encourage your children to listen, look, smell (and, when appropriate, taste and feel) the natural world around them. Just remember—follow safety guidelines and Leave No Trace ethics and put back anything you find!

Fens and bogs are nutrient-poor, acidic, peat-accumulating wetlands. Home to sphagnum moss, evergreen shrubs, and sedges, fens and bogs also provide habitat for mammals such as moose and beavers, as well as for nesting shorebirds.

Marshes are wetlands dominated by grasses, rushes, and reeds and found at the edges of streams and lakes; **swamps** are wetlands dominated by trees. Both provide critical habitat for a diversity of invertebrates, amphibians, waterfowl, fish, and aquatic mammals. **Vernal pools** are marshes found only seasonally in shallow depressions, creating temporary pool ecosystems in forested landscapes.

Flowing water habitats include everything from seeps, springs, and streams to raging rivers and gushing waterfalls. Streams and rivers provide shelter and feeding opportunities for a vast range of plants and animals.

A classic distinction between **ponds** and **lakes** is that sunlight penetrates to the bottom of all areas of a pond, whereas it will not in a lake's deeper waters. Lakes are generally larger in surface area, too, but both provide critical habitat for aquatic invertebrates, plankton, fish, wildlife, and vegetation.

The most common **grassland habitats** here are agricultural fields where vegetation consists of a mixture of grasses, sedges, and wildflowers. More than 70 species of wildlife use these open areas for breeding grounds, cover, or food, including songbirds, small rodents, white-tailed deer, snakes, and frogs.

Our mosaic of **forest habitats** includes boreal spruce-fir forests to the north and deciduous forests to the south. Some combination of sugar maple, American beech, and yellow birch characterize most hardwood forests, while mixed forests of spruce, balsam fir, red pine, eastern hemlock, and eastern white pine are also present. Characteristic mammals include black bears, red foxes, porcupines, beavers, muskrats, raccoons, and white-tailed deer.

Trees can often provide more wildlife habitats when they're dead than alive. Birds, small mammals, and other wildlife use standing dead and dying trees—called "snags"—for nests, foraging, roosting, and perching. Live trees provide similar value to wildlife via snag-like features such as hollow trunks, dead branches, and excavated cavities.

Look for these common New England animals and plants when you're outside, and bring a field guide along on your next adventure!

Animals

- Black bears
- Moose
- White-tailed deer
- Beavers
- Otters
- Mice
- Chipmunks
- Rabbits
- Squirrels
- Foxes
- Raccoons
- Weasels
- Muskrats
- Tree frogs
- Bullfrogs
- Lizards
- Snakes

Wildflowers

- Trillium
- Bunchberry
- Pink lady's slipper
- Blue-bead lily
- Pitcher plant
- Sundew

Trip 15

Carriage Roads

Close to nature and free from motorized vehicles, Acadia's wide, broken-stone roads traverse impressive granite bridges and blend with the landscape, highlighting the stunning scenery.

Address: Duck Brook Road (between Eagle Lake Road and West Street Extension), Bar Harbor
Difficulty: Easy–Moderate
Distance: 3.3–10.0 miles, round-trip
Hours: No posted hours; contact park for seasonal road and trail closures
Fee: $20 per vehicle; $5 per adult without a vehicle, including bicyclists and pedestrians (children under 15 are free)
Contact: Acadia National Park, 207-288-3338, nps.gov/acad; Island Explorer Bike Express, 207 667 5796, exploreacadia.com/bikeexpress.htm
Bathrooms: At the parking area on the north end of Eagle Lake and at park headquarters
Water/Snacks: None
Maps: USGS Southwest Harbor and Bar Harbor quads; *Acadia National Park Discovery Map* (AMC), Eastern Mount Desert Island: B6–D6
Directions by Car: From the junction of ME 3 and ME 233 in Bar Harbor, head west on ME 233/Eagle Lake Road for 2.0 miles. Turn right onto Duck Brook Road, passing a beaver dam on New Mill Meadow. Park your vehicle at the roadside parking area near the bridge. The carriage road intersects the road here at numbered intersection signpost #5 (44° 23.467′ N, 68° 14.130′ W).
Directions by Bus: From late June through Columbus Day, ride the fare-free Island Explorer Bike Express bus to the carriage roads. More information is available online, at the Hulls Cove Visitor Center, and at park headquarters.

When John D. Rockefeller Jr. designed the 45 miles of carriage trails in Acadia National Park in the early 1900s, he had one primary goal: showcase the natural splendor of the area for visitors traveling by horse-drawn carriage. The roads follow the land's contours so that waterfalls can be seen from either direction and scenic viewpoints come into focus at every turn. Instead of bypassing streams all together, Rockefeller commissioned sixteen beautiful granite bridges. Today, the broken-stone carriage roads are well maintained by the Friends of Acadia and serve bikes, horses, and pedestrians. When biking

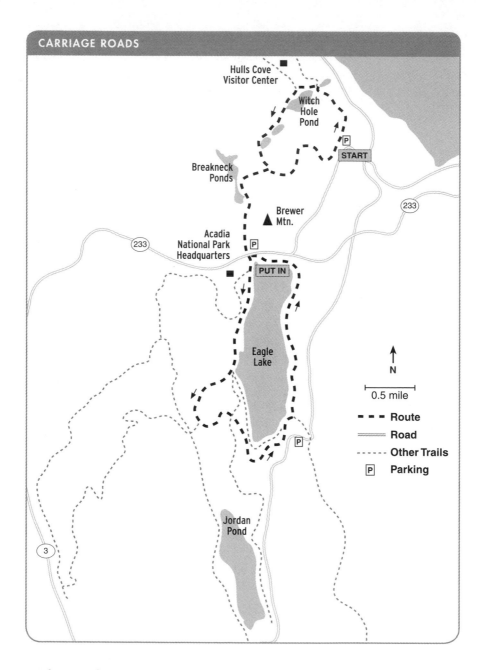

Hulls Cove
Visitor Center

Witch
Hole
Pond

P

START

Breakneck
Ponds

Brewer
Mtn.

233

Acadia
National Park
Headquarters

233

P

PUT IN

Eagle
Lake

N

0.5 mile

Route

Road

Other Trails

P   Parking

Jordan
Pond

3

on this or other carriage roads in the park, hybrid or mountain bikes are recommended. Also, keep in mind that the carriage roads are not one-way streets;
feel free to turn around and retrace your steps at any point.

Begin this 3.3-mile, family-friendly, counterclockwise loop around Witch
Hole Pond from Duck Brook Road at signpost #5. All carriage road intersections are numbered on these wooden posts. Head to the right (northeast).

Though the trail initially climbs for approximately 100 feet, it soon levels out. One mile after beginning, reach signpost #3 and take a left. Here, up-close views of Witch Hole Pond come into focus. Continue making your way along the pond, bearing left at signpost #2. At mile 2.3, reach signpost #4. At this point, assess the stamina and interest of your group. If the kids are getting tired, bear left here, continuing for 1.0 mile to signpost #5, where you began. If you and yours feel like your legs are just warming up, consider adding another 6.7 miles to your route by circumnavigating Eagle Lake, too. Though the Eagle Lake loop does have more challenging, hilly terrain, it is considered one of the most beautiful rides within the park.

To continue to Eagle Lake, turn right at signpost #4. Enjoy the views of Halfmoon Pond on the 1.1-mile stretch to signpost #6. Continue under a bridge and pass close by the Eagle Lake parking area. Stay right (bearing southwest) here and reach signpost #9. The carriage road continues along the western side of Eagle Lake. Be prepared for some hilly terrain between signposts #9 and #8, which you will reach in 5.5 miles. After taking a rest here, continue left (heading east) as the carriage road continues along the southern flank of Eagle Lake. At signpost #7, bear left to follow the eastern side of the lake northward and make your way back toward signpost #6. Bear right at signpost #6, travel the 1.1 miles north to signpost #4, then take a right to travel 1.0 mile back to signpost #5 where you began.

PLAN B: Traditional sightseeing carriage rides are available on the carriage roads from a concession located at Acadia's Wildwood Stables. Because the rides are very popular during peak season, advance reservations are highly recommended. For more information, visit Hulls Cove Visitor Center or park headquarters.

NEARBY: After burning through calories on your bicycle, what's better than a popover and some lobster bisque? The Jordan Pond House, Acadia National Park's only full-service restaurant, is a popular destination among visitors (thejordanpondhouse.com). Nearby, the bustling town of Bar Harbor offers a full range of restaurants, cafés, ice cream shops, and more.

Consider a visit to one of the area's many museums, including Acadia's Sieur de Monts Spring and Nature Center, located on Park Loop Road. It offers hands-on exhibits to learn about the area's plants and animals. Farther afield, check out the Mount Desert Oceanarium, where you can get up-close-and-personal with marine life. The Oceanarium offers marsh tours, a lobster hatchery, and the Discovery Pool Touch Tank (theoceanarium.com).

Trip 16

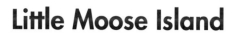

Little Moose Island

Cross a land bridge to this 54-acre island teeming with wildlife (not with Acadia's usual crowds) and bordered by a loop trail with stunning coastal views.

Address: East Schoodic Drive, Gouldsboro
Difficulty: Easy–Moderate
Distance: 1.6 miles round-trip
Hours: No posted hours; contact park for seasonal road and trail closures
Fee: $20 per vehicle; $5 per adult without a vehicle, including bicyclists and pedestrians (children under 15 are free)
Contact: Acadia National Park, 207-288-3338, nps.gov/acad; Island Explorer Bike Express, 207-667-5796, exploreacadia.com/bikeexpress.htm
Bathrooms: At nearby Frazer Point
Water/Snacks: Water fountain at nearby Frazer Point
Maps: USGS Schoodic Head quad; *Acadia National Park Discovery Map* (AMC), Schoodic Peninsula
Directions by Car: From Ellsworth, take US 1 east. In 19.0 miles, turn right and travel right on US 186 for approximately 6.0 miles. Turn right off Main Street at the National Park sign for Schoodic Peninsula. The road becomes a one-way park loop after 1.0 mile. Continue past the sign for Schoodic Point (a great place to stop for spectacular coastal views) for approximately 0.75 mile to the small turnout and unmarked parking area on your right, adjacent to Little Moose Island. A short trail leads from there down to the land bridge, which you can cross at low tide to access the island trailhead (44° 20.201′ N, 68° 3.080′ W). Consult a tidal chart before this journey to ensure passage back to mainland before the tide rises!
Directions by Bus: From late June through Columbus Day, ride the fare-free Island Explorer Bike Express bus to the Schoodic section of the park. More information is available online, at the Hulls Cove Visitor Center, and at park headquarters.

Located on the southeastern tip of Schoodic Peninsula, 54-acre Little Moose Island is a part of Acadia National Park, though you won't encounter the droves of tourists here that descend on nearby Mount Desert Island. Instead, you'll find droves of wildlife and an adventurous island hike that kids of all ages will enjoy.

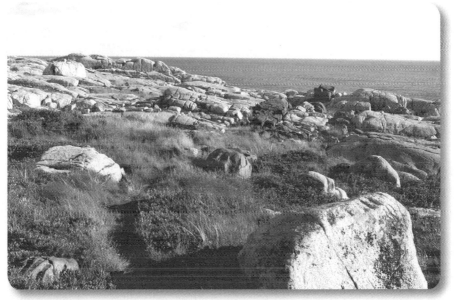

Dramatic coastal scenery is just one highlight of a hike on Little Moose Island.

The biggest challenge (and greatest attraction) about this hike is that it can be completed only during low tide when the land bridge connecting Little Moose Island and the mainland is accessible. Be sure to consult a tidal map when planning this hike to ensure that you won't be stranded on the island, waiting for the next low tide. Tidal knowledge is important when traveling the coast of Maine, so this hike offers a great opportunity to talk with your children about tides and what creates them. Because of the earth's rotation and the moon's rotation, high tide lasts approximately 6 hours and low tide lasts approximately 6 hours. Given that information and a little advance planning, you will have plenty of time to explore Little Moose Island on foot.

The first part of your journey to Little Moose involves crossing the intertidal zone between the mainland and island. Watch your footing on the slippery rocks, which are covered with dense bundles of Irish moss and seaweed known as rockweed or bladderwrack (easily recognized by its air-filled "bladders" that keep the plant afloat). Take it slow here, pausing to see how many of the 40 species of the intertidal zone's invertebrates you can find, including crabs and seastars.

Cross the beach on the western side of the island and make your way toward the trailhead, which begins on the island's northwest corner, marked with a small interpretive sign describing the fragile inland vegetation and requesting that hikers stay on trail. The trail crosses weather-battered rock that will delight budding geologists: notice the striking feature of black, basalt dikes that cut through pale pink granite. Continue on the fairly level trail, through shrubby land dotted with wild blueberries (in season), beach roses, laurel, yarrow, cow parsnip, and sea lavender. The vibrant pink and purple flowers contrast with the greens of the inland forest and blues of the ocean and sky to make for a dazzling array of color. This is coastal Maine at its finest. The trail eventually leads to the southern tip of the island where you'll be compelled to break for a while and take in the astounding scenery and plentiful seabirds before turning back and retracing your steps toward the trailhead.

PLAN B: The 6.0-mile Schoodic Loop Road (one-way traffic) offers views of lighthouses, seabirds, and forest-draped islands. Turnouts provide opportunities to pull over and enjoy the views. An unpaved road leads to the top of 400-foot-high Schoodic Head and its spectacular views of Frenchman Bay and Mount Desert Island, including Cadillac Mountain. Or, hike up Schoodic in 0.6 mile via Schoodic Head Trail, which connects with the other three trails within the area—Anvil Trail (1.1 miles), East Trail (0.5 mile), and Alder Trail (0.6 mile)—all of which have trailheads off of Schoodic Loop Road. Additional camping and bicycling opportunities exist at Schoodic Woods; for more information, visit schoodicwoods.com.

NEARBY: When visiting the Schoodic Peninsula, be sure to check out the unique, unspoiled fishing villages in the area, such as Corea, Prospect Harbor, and Winter Harbor. During the summer months, a ferry service provides transportation from Winter Harbor to Bar Harbor. Contact 207-288-2984 for additional ferry information.

MORE KID-FRIENDLY TRIPS ELSEWHERE IN ACADIA
Looking for more trails while you're in Acadia? Try these:
- Cadillac Summit Loop Trail (0.5 miles)
- Beech Cliff Trail (0.8 miles)
- Wonderland Trail (1.4 miles)
- Gorham Mountain Trail (3.0 miles)
- Ocean Path (3.0 miles)

Inland Maine

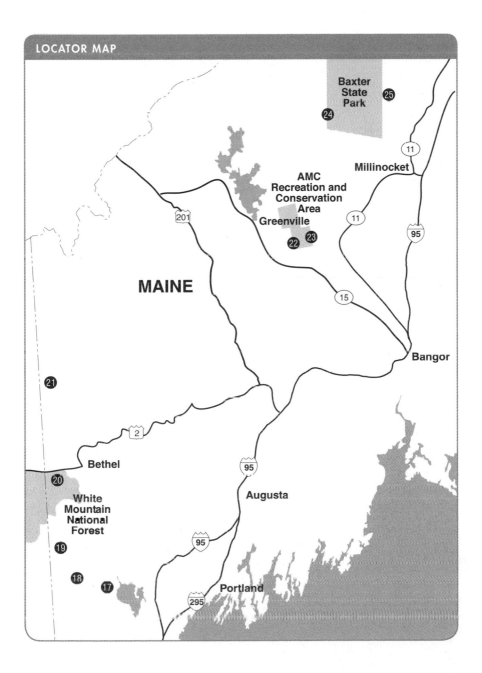

LOCATOR MAP

Baxter State Park

25

24

11

Millinocket

AMC Recreation and Conservation Area

Greenville

201

11

95

22

23

15

MAINE

Bangor

21

2

Bethel

95

20

White Mountain National Forest

Augusta

19

95

18

17

Portland

295

Trip 17

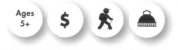

Ages 5+

Douglas Mountain

A stone observation tower from the 1920s offers great views toward the White Mountains and Sebago Lake.

Address: Douglas Mountain Road, Sebago
Difficulty: Moderate
Distance: 1.25 miles, loop
Hours: Sunrise to sunset
Fee: $3 suggested donation per vehicle
Contact: Town of Sebago, 207-787-2457, townofsebago.org/Pages/SebagoME_DPW/dgm.jpg
Bathrooms: Portable toilet at trailhead
Water/Snacks: None
Maps: USGS Steep Falls quad; townofsebago.org/Pages/SebagoME_DPW/dgm.jpg
Directions by Car: Follow ME 107 north for 5.6 miles from East Baldwin or south 10.0 miles from Bridgton. Turn on to Dyke Mountain Road. In 0.8 mile, turn left onto Douglas Mountain Road and follow signs for the parking area (43° 52.305′ N, 70° 41.787′ W) and trailheads. The primary trailhead begins from the parking area; the second trailhead is located 0.2 mile farther up Douglas Mountain Road and is for drop-off/pick-up only.

A large boulder on the Douglas Mountain summit bears the inscription *non sibi sed omnibus*, a Latin motto meaning "not for one, but for all." This 169-acre preserve was deeded to the town of Sebago by The Nature Conservancy in 1996. The 16-foot stone observation tower at the top adds an enticing feature to this family-friendly hike, which is less than an hour's drive from downtown Portland. Note that hunting is allowed on Douglas Mountain in season. Wear blaze orange from October through December to ensure that you are seen.

From the well-marked parking area, take orange-blazed Eagle Scout Trail, which (aptly) was blazed by a group of Eagle Scouts. For the majority of the way, this trail closely follows or shares a wide, moderately hilly snowmobile trail. During wetter months, prepare to cross a few small streams as you venture through the forested lowlands. At approximately 0.75 mile, Eagle Scout Trail splits from the wider snowmobile trail, narrows, and proceeds at a steeper

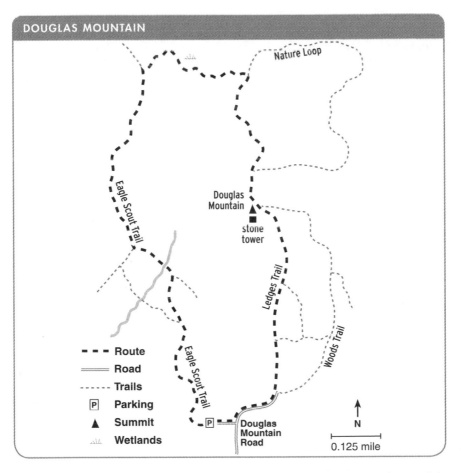

pitch toward the summit. Watch your feet in areas, avoiding exposed roots, but be sure to pay close attention to the orange blazes.

On the wide summit (1.0 mile), kids will be running for the stone tower. It was built in 1925 by three local men, including Harry E. Douglas, who inspired the mountain's name. Douglas used his oxen to haul up the materials used to construct the sturdy lookout. Climbing up the stone steps through the structure to its observation platform feels somewhat like ascending the turret of an ancient castle. From the platform, you can see a fantastic view of Sebago Lake and, in the distance, the White Mountains.

Descend via 0.25-mile Ledges Trail. Look for the trail marker at the southwestern edge of the open summit, then follow the yellow blazes down to the drop-off point on Douglas Mountain Road. From there, it's a short walk along the road back to the parking area where you started.

PLAN B: Nearby Sebago Lake is a popular destination thanks to its crystal clear water, great views, and beaches. It's the deepest lake in New England, holding almost a trillion gallons of water. And it's so exceptionally clean that it is exempt from needing filtration equipment to convert it to drinking water.

You can also head to Sebago Lake State Park, a 1,400-acre protected area featuring sandy beaches, woodlands, ponds, bogs, a river, and plenty of trails.

NEARBY: For amenities, head north to the small town of Bridgton, home to Pondicherry Park, which features walking trails, boardwalks, an educational amphitheater and two beautiful bridges spanning the brooks (mainelakes. org/?page_id=1028).

Trip 18

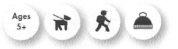

Burnt Meadow Mountain

Gain elevation and stunning views quickly on this relatively strenuous trail, great for kids who aren't afraid to climb!

Address: ME 160/Spring Road, Brownfield
Difficulty: Moderate–Challenging
Distance: 2.6 miles, round-trip
Hours: Sunrise to sunset
Fee: Free
Contact: Friends of Burnt Meadow Mountains,
    friendsofburntmeadowmountains.com
Bathrooms: None
Water/Snacks: None
Maps: USGS Brownfield quad; friendsofburntmeadowmountains.com/graphic_
    html-links/bmm_trail_map.html
Directions by Car: From the junction of US 302 and ME 5/ME 113 in Fryeburg,
    take ME 5/ME 113 heading south to Brownfield. In 6.9 miles, turn right onto
    ME 160 South. In 3.0 miles (approximately 0.5 mile south of the pond),
    there is an unmarked but obvious parking area on the right (43° 55.126′ N,
    70° 52.753′ W).

If your kids are bored with introductory hikes and up for a little adventure, including a rocky scramble near the summit, head to Burnt Meadow Mountain. The mountain's name comes from its tragic history. In October 1947, small, localized fires from Mount Desert Island to Waterboro morphed into one statewide disaster, burning more than 200,000 acres over a short period becoming known collectively as "the week that Maine burned." Here, a great forest fire incinerated an estimated 85 percent of the town of Brownfield and the surrounding area, including this mountain. Today it's hard to see evidence of the fire (or the ski area that had a short-lived run here in the 1970s), as nature has taken back its own.

What you do see in the sweeping views from the summit is majestic forest that seems to go on and on, broken only by myriad ponds and distant mountains, including those of the Presidential Range. The North Peak summit is broad and grassy, offering plenty of room to spread out and relax. During the

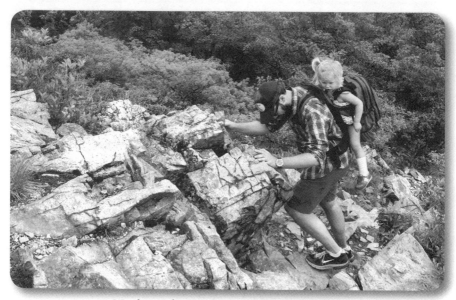

Watch your feet over loose rocks on the final pitch toward the summit of Burnt Meadow Mountain.

late summer, blueberries and red mountain cranberries dot the landscape. Autumn is an excellent time to visit as well: the summit views of fall foliage are out of this world.

From the parking area, North Peak Trail (Burnt Meadow Trail) begins on the right and takes the shortest and most rewarding—albeit steepest—trek to the summit. The blue-blazed trail is well marked as soon as you enter into the forest. Expansive views southeast greet you before you've hiked even 0.25 mile. The trail meanders up through the woodlands, occasionally bringing you to exposed ledges where you can catch glimpses of nearby mountains, including Pleasant Mountain (Trip 19) to the north and the two other peaks of Burnt Meadow Mountain to the southwest. The first 0.5 mile is the best terrain for younger hikers, as the pitch gets steeper after that; parents should be prepared to carry preschoolers.

At 0.7 mile, the trail opens onto an exposed ledge with an excellent view. Look for Burnt Meadow Pond below and the North Peak summit above. If the scramble that awaits you above seems too daunting for your party, this could be an excellent place to stop, have a picnic lunch, and turn around for home. However, if kids are feeling strong and ambitious, continue onward and up-ward. Just past 1.1 miles, the scramble begins in earnest; watch your feet over loose rocks and make sure your handholds are steady. Kids of any age will need help—and perhaps a hand now and then—as they make their way up the final pitches toward the summit.

Once at North Peak, take a moment to congratulate everyone for making it up 1,200 vertical feet in just 1.3 miles—that's no easy feat! You will all take pride in the accomplishment, particularly when you're treated with majestic 360-degree views.

To descend, retrace your steps down the mountain via North Peak Trail. If that seems too treacherous, opt for longer, more gradual Twin Brook Trail, which you'll see marked with yellow blazes. This 2.0-mile trail follows the main brook and ravine before eventually meeting back up with North Peak Trail near the trailhead.

PLAN B: The White Mountain National Forest offers a plethora of swimming holes, hikes, and beaches, many of which are a half-hour drive from Burnt Meadow Mountain (see Trips 35 and 36). For more information, visit www. fs.usda.gov/whitemountain.

NEARBY: Head to the quintessential New England village of North Conway, New Hampshire, 20 miles to the west, where historic buildings, bookstores, bakeries, and big-name outlet stores all coexist. North Conway is the gateway to the White Mountain National Forest and also home to Mount Washington Valley Children's Museum (mwvchildrensmuseum.org; 603-356-2992).

Trip 19

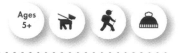

Pleasant Mountain

With stunning views of lakes and mountains, it's no wonder how southern Maine's tallest peak earned its name.

Address: Denmark Road (between West Denmark Road and Spiked Ridge Drive), Denmark
Difficulty: Moderate
Distance: 3.4–5.8 miles, round-trip
Hours: No posted hours
Fee: Free
Contact: Loon Echo Land Trust, 207-647-4352, loonecholandtrust.org/places-we-protect/preserves/pleasant-mountain-preserve
Bathrooms: None
Water/Snacks: None
Maps: USGS Pleasant Mountain quad; *AMC Maine Mountain Guide*, 10th edition (AMC); *Maine Atlas and Gazetteer*, Map 4 (DeLorme); loonecholandtrust.org/wp-content/uploads/2014/01/lelt_pleasant-mtn_map_rev2013-final.pdf
Directions by Car: From downtown Bridgton continue on US 302 for approximately 8.3 miles. Turn left onto Wilton Warren Road, follow it to its end at Denmark Road, and turn left. In 0.4 mile, bear left at the Y onto Rocky Knoll Road/Denmark Road. Continue for another 0.4 miles to the unmarked parking area on your left (44° 6.155′ N, 70° 52.107′ W), across from Spiked Ridge Drive.

At 2,006 feet, Pleasant Mountain is southern Maine's tallest mountain, home to Shawnee Peak Ski Area and a 10-mile trail network offering an array of terrain. This route on Southwest Ridge Trail is a moderately strenuous, family-friendly hike that will leave everyone with a great sense of accomplishment.

From the well-marked trailhead, the wide, compacted dirt path ascends gradually at first through mixed forest for 0.6 mile, where it gains the ridge. From here, the trail weaves its way upward, alternating between slab granite and compact dirt. The views to the southeast get more and more stunning with each step. Moose Pond, the largest nearby body of water, glistens below (see Plan B).

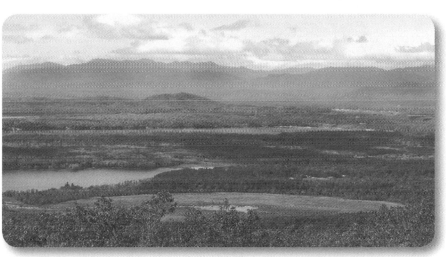

Southwest Ridge Trail offers stunning views of the southern Lakes Region and beyond.

The trail rises moderately along the exposed ridge, marked along the way with yellow blazes and rock cairns. Make sure your family is well prepared for the elements, whether it's a warm, sunny day or a cool, wet one. Plentiful fields of wild blueberries thrive in this open habitat and (in season) provide the perfect sweet snack to fuel your climb.

After hiking 1.7 miles and gaining 1,546 feet in elevation, reach the Southwest Summit and take in the sweeping views of the southern Lakes Region. Most families will want to turn around here and retrace their steps back to the trailhead; however, if you have the energy and desire to push onward, consider hiking another 1.2 miles to the main summit. This additional route passes a small fire tower and a wide-open rocky field with superb views of western Maine and the White Mountains of New Hampshire.

PLAN B: Moose Pond's calm waters, stunning scenery, abundant wildlife, and coves ripe for exploration make it an ideal body of water for family canoe trips. The 11-mile-long pond is divided into three distinct basins—the southernmost one being the most protected. From US 302 and Wilton Warren Road, take US 302 east for 2.8 miles to the causeway/bridge that separates the two largest basins of Moose Pond. The public boat launch is on the left. For canoe rentals, contact Shawnee Peak Ski Area (207-647-8444).

NEARBY: Bridgton offers shopping, restaurants, an arts community, and a movie theater. North Conway, New Hampshire, is 15 miles away.

Trip 20

All Ages $ 🐕   🚶

The Roost

Hike a half-mile in Evans Notch along a moderate trail to reach great views of the Wild River Valley and White Mountains.

Address: Wild River Road, Gilead
Difficulty: Easy–Moderate
Distance: 1.0 mile, round-trip
Hours: No posted hours
Fee: $3 daily pass per vehicle
Contact: White Mountain National Forest, 603-535-6100,
  www.fs.usda.gov/whitemountain
Bathrooms: None
Water/Snacks: None
Maps: USGS Speckled Mountain quad; *Maine Mountains Trail Map*,
  Map 7: E13 (AMC)
Directions by Car: From the junction of US 2 and ME 113 in Gilead, head south on ME 113 for 2.9 miles. The Roost trailhead is on the left, with minimal parking available along the road (44° 20.339′ N, 70° 59.446′ W). Additional parking is available 100 yards ahead, across the bridge.

Aside from the first steep 50 feet and the last 100 feet, the grade on this moderately inclined trail makes it a family favorite. There are few other trails in Maine's western mountains where you can access such spectacular views after hiking only 0.5 mile. It's short and moderate enough that little kids can do it. Bigger kids will like the fact that they can race to the top to access great views, especially since the trail is well established, marked with yellow blazes, and uninterrupted by spur trails or junctions. And everyone will enjoy ample blueberries or stunning fall foliage in their respective seasons.

From the trailhead, you must first contend with a short but steep set of rock stairs. Don't fret: this is the most arduous part of the trail, and you approach it right out of the gate! Beyond the stairs, the path winds comfortably uphill through lowland forest, including a stand of handsome paper birches.

Just 0.25 mile from the trailhead, the trail crosses a trickling stream that may entice little hikers with its frogs, wiggly insects, and streamside mushrooms of all different colors. Continue up trail to the summit (0.5 miles from

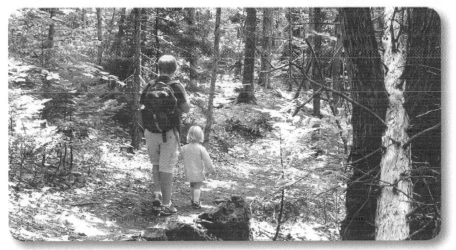
Kids big and small will enjoy the short hike to The Roost in Evans Notch.

the trailhead), which is an exposed bald face bordered with pines, hemlocks, and spruces. A sign indicates that you've reached The Roost, though take note that scenic views are better farther along.

Bearing right onto a side trail from the bald face, follow the arrow shown on a Scenic View sign. The path descends a few hundred feet through the forest before it opens onto a spectacular overlook where there is plenty of room to spread out a picnic lunch, kick up your heels, and take in the scenery. The Wild River Valley spreads below while East Royce Mountain rises in the southwest and other White Mountain peaks stud the landscape to the west. Once you've taken in the sights (and as many blueberries as you can during the late summer months), retrace your steps to return to the trailhead.

PLAN B: The Evans Notch area of the White Mountain National Forest has a number of family-friendly hikes, including 3.2-mile East Royce Trail, 4-mile Albany Mountain Trail, and 4.6-mile Basic Trail to Rim Junction. To find out more about any of these hikes, contact the White Mountain National Forest.

Nearby Bethel, "Maine's Most Beautiful Mountain Village," serves as gateway to the Androscoggin River, a popular destination for canoeing, kayaking, or tubing adventures. The Bethel Pathway is a 3-mile round-trip, paved, wheelchair-accessible trail winding along the Androscoggin; it can be accessed from a parking lot on ME 2 or at Davis Park on ME 26, where there is also a picnic area, skate park, and playground.

NEARBY: Bethel offers a number of small diners, coffee shops, and markets where you can pick up provisions or sit down for an enjoyable meal.

Trip 21

Table Rock

Spectacular views await after either a moderate one-way hike or a more challenging loop up chutes and ladders in the scenic Grafton Notch area.

Address: ME 26 (between Bean Put Hill and York Town Road), Newry
Difficulty: Moderate
Distance: 2.4–3.0 miles, round-trip
Hours: No posted hours
Fee: $2 adult Maine residents, $3 adult nonresidents, $1 children ages 5–11
Contact: Grafton Notch State Park, 207-824-2912, parksandlands.com
Bathrooms: Rustic restrooms at trailhead
Water/Snacks: None
Maps: USGS Old Speck Mountain quad; *AMC Mahoosucs Map & Guide*, E5 (AMC)
Directions by Car: From the junction of US 2/ME 5 and ME 26 in Bethel, drive north on ME 26 for 12.0 miles to a large off-road parking area for Old Speck Mountain on the left (44° 35.383′ N 70° 56.801′ W).

Grafton Notch is one of Maine's most spectacular recreational areas, rife with cascading waters, swimming holes, mountain peaks, and abundant trails. Backcountry terrain here can be rugged, and the 3,000-acre state park includes twelve of the most challenging miles along the whole Appalachian Trail (AT). This hike to Table Rock balances a taste of rugged backcountry adventure with family-friendly manageability.

The trailhead begins from the northern side of the parking lot. Take the white-blazed AT to your right, which leads briefly into the forest before crossing over ME 26. Cars often travel quickly over this winding road, so proceed cautiously. The trail picks up on the other side, marked by a brown sign of a hiker with a walking stick. Kids will enjoy balancing on the halved-log boardwalk that keeps them elevated from the soggy terrain below. After just over 0.1 mile of trekking though woodlands, the trail reaches a prominent junction. To the right, the orange-blazed, 1.3-mile Table Rock Trail beckons. Only experienced hikers and older children should attempt this trail, as it rises steeply through a series of tricky chutes and ladders and crosses potentially

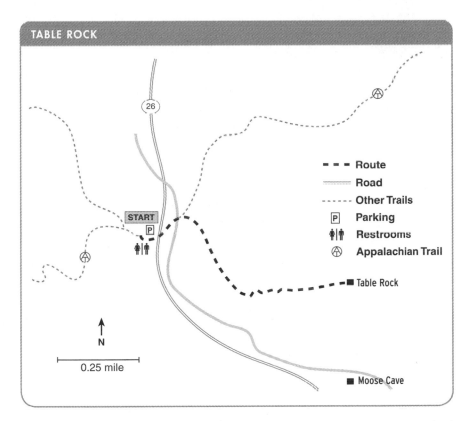

TABLE ROCK

Legend:
- - - Route
——— Road
------ Other Trails
P Parking
♦♦ Restrooms
Ⓐ Appalachian Trail
■ Table Rock

26

START
P
♦♦

N

0.25 mile

■ Moose Cave

treacherous boulder fields on its way to the summit. The route as described here is a tamer adventure: bear left at the trail junction, following the white-blaze AT.

You are likely to share this section of trail with sure-footed hikers loaded with big backpacks—particularly if you're hiking in late summer and fall. Many of these travelers are part of an elite group of adventurers who hike the whole 2,000-mile AT from Springer Mountain, Georgia, to the top of Katahdin. Most "thru-hikers" appreciate a word of encouragement and congratulations (not to mention any fresh food you feel like sharing), so don't be afraid to say hello.

The wide, rugged trail rises at a moderate grade through the forest, crossing a stream at just over 0.3 mile before briefly leveling. At approximately 1.0 mile, it reaches a second trail junction. Bear right (south) onto the blue-blazed trail at a sign for Table Rock, leaving the AT behind. The ascent is moderate most of the way to the summit (1.5 miles), save for the final few hundred feet, which is steep.

The large, flat summit juts out over its supporting base like a tabletop, offering a spectacular perch. On a clear day look for mountains in the Mahoosuc Range, including Puzzle Mountain, Old Speck, and Sunday River Whitecap.

The granite slab is the perfect setting for lunch—just be sure kids sit far enough from the ledge, as the drop-off is extreme.

To descend, choose one of two options: retrace your steps down the moderate blue-blazed trail and the AT for a 3.0-mile round-trip, or create a loop via the challenging orange-blazed Table Rock Trail. If choosing the latter, be sure your whole group is prepared to descend down steep, rocky terrain that tests even the most sure-footed hikers (and rewards them with exciting features and plenty of great views).

The trail meets the summit at its northeastern corner before plunging down through woods into a gully. Keep your eye on the orange blazes, which are prominently placed to mark the way. At 0.1 mile, pass below the ledges supporting Table Rock before tracing the narrow path through massive boulders and alongside slab caves that are sure to delight hikers old and young. The rocky jungle requires patience and attention, though kids will likely revel in the challenge.

After picking through the boulder field, enjoy the views of Old Speck Mountain looming in front of you. The trail then leads down an impressive series of rock steps, stairways, and drainage devices installed by the Maine Conservation Corps over the course of four years. Can kids imagine how much sweat went into carrying and placing all those rocks?!

Eventually, the steep grade becomes more gradual and, at 1.3 miles from Table Rock, reunites with the white-blazed AT. Turn left at this junction, continuing back to the trailhead.

PLAN B: Grafton Notch offers a plethora of highlights, including one of Maine's most heavily visited waterfalls, Screw Auger Falls. The 23-foot cascade is located 1.0 mile north of the Grafton Notch State Park entrance and accessible via an easy 0.1-mile jaunt off ME 26 from the large parking area (complete with picnic tables and bathrooms), and it's easy to see why crowds are drawn here. It plunges over the lip of a broad granite ledge into a narrow gorge. Below the waterfall, the Bear River drops in a series of cascades through interesting terrain, including large potholes, grottoes, and shallow pools. Explore above and below the falls, but exercise caution: there are many ledges and drop-offs.

Other nearby destinations include the kid-friendly Mother Walker Falls, which is located 1.1 miles north of Screw Auger Falls and similarly offers an easily-accessible waterfall that roars over broken rocks, eventually descending nearly 100 feet. The 200-foot-long Moose Cave is another popular destination, as are Step Falls and Spruce Meadow Picnic Area, which boasts spectacular views of Old Speck Mountain and overlooks a wildlife-rich marsh.

Wherever you go in Grafton Notch, be on the lookout for birds: the state park is a part of the Maine Birding Trail and a popular destination for those looking to observe peregrine falcons, a wide variety of songbirds, and even some Northern Forest species at high elevations.

NEARBY: The scenic, quaint mountain town of Bethel (less than a half hour's drive from Grafton Notch State Park) offers a number of small diners, coffee shops, and markets where you can pick up provisions or sit down for an enjoyable meal.

Let's face it—sometimes kids just don't want to hike or paddle or pedal. They may be tired; the hill might be steep; the weather may be hot. Traveling in the outdoors can be hard work for children and downright unenjoyable if they feel they are on a forced march. You will find that on occasion, the kids will just stop. That's when you need games on the move!

When you sense attention spans and patience beginning to wane, try out these games before you throw in the towel and head back to the car. Chances are they may enable you and the family to happily keep moving toward your destination!

Essence

One person thinks of a person that everyone in the group knows. The other players try to guess the identity of the person, but unlike Twenty Questions, all questions must follow this format: "If this person were a _____, what type of _____ would they be?" Fill in the blank and ask what type of car, food, weather, city, geographic feature, or animal the subject would be. Sometimes the first couple of answers give away the subject's identity, so we always have a rule that you must ask at least five questions before guessing the answer.

Candy Forest

This game is simple and effective, especially with younger kids. One adult goes ahead on the trail and hides colorful snacks in obvious hiding places along the trail: in the crook of a small tree, in a rock crack, or on a trail sign. Space them over a few hundred yards, then a new player gets to hide the treats.

Tree Huggers

This game is kind of like hiking Musical Chairs, with a chance to identify trees thrown in. One person serves as the Tree Master. As you are hiking, the Tree Master calls out the name of a tree, such as an oak. Everyone then has to run and hug an oak tree. Last one to hug an oak is out. Continue until only one person remains—that's your new Tree Master!

ABCs

Starting with the letter A, everyone has to find something along the trail or river that begins with A, then move through the rest of the alphabet.

Roving Hide and Seek

This is best played with slightly older kids who you aren't worried will wander off the trail on their own. One player (the hider) runs ahead on the trail and finds a tree, rock, or object to hide behind or under, ideally within 10–15 feet of the trail. The rest of the group can keep hiking (slowly) while the hider runs ahead. The fun of the game is that the hider gets to jump out and startle the seekers as they hike along the trail—just be sure that you surprise your own group and not unsuspecting strangers! Rotate hiders so everyone gets a chance—adults included!

Trail Bingo

Everyone picks one object that you are likely to see on the trail. Examples on a hike might be a stream, a hiker with blue shorts, a squirrel, and a red backpack. After everyone has chosen an object, you begin to play.

The game works like bingo—everyone is looking to find the objects you chose, but only one person can claim each sighting.

If you come across a hiker wearing blue shorts (or a squirrel or a stream, etc.), the player who sees the object first should say "BINGO: Blue shorts!" You must say BINGO first! Now, no one else can claim those blue shorts—they must find their own.

If you find a group of something (like a group of several squirrels), that sighting counts only as one squirrel. Only one person can claim squirrels; everyone else must find another squirrel (or group of squirrels). The first person to find all of the objects that the group chose (and calls BINGO for each one), wins!

This works really well in the car as well. Police cars, boats, animals, and ice cream stands are popular options, but the objects you can choose are limitless! Make sure the objects you choose are not too rare or too common. If you are trying to find a tree while on a hike, the game will be instantly over. Try finding a birch tree or a fallen tree, instead.

Categories

Think of a specific category such as state capitals, colored foods, countries that begin with M, or sports teams. Everyone takes turns naming something that fits in that category. Play rotates through the group until someone can't think of something (in 5 seconds) or until a name gets repeated.

Trip 22

Borestone Mountain Audubon Sanctuary

Hike through old forest to a seasonal pond-side nature center and scramble to a baldface summit with 360-degree views of the 100-Mile Wilderness.

Address: Mountain Road (between Elliottsville Road and Bodfish Valley Road), Monson
Difficulty: Moderate–Challenging
Distance: 1.6–3.6 miles, round-trip
Hours: Dawn to dusk
Fee: $5 nonmembers over 6; free for Audubon Society members
Contact: Maine Audubon, 207-631-4050 (June–September), 207-781-2330 (October–May), maineaudubon.org/find-us/borestone-mountain-sanctuary/
Bathrooms: Up the trail 0.8 mile
Water/Snacks: None
Maps: USGS Barren Mountain West quad; mainetrailfinder.com/trails/trail/borestone-mountain-audubon-sanctuary; *Maine Atlas and Gazetteer*, Map 41 (DeLorme)
Directions by Car: From ME 6/15 and Elliotsville Road in Monson, turn right (north) onto Elliotsville Road, which is marked by an Audubon Society sign. Drive 8.0 miles, crossing Wilson Stream, and bear left onto Bodfish Road after the bridge. Proceed uphill for 0.2 mile, across railroad tracks, to the parking area on your left. The gate to the sanctuary and trailhead is on the right (45° 24.534′ N, 69° 23.608′ W).

Borestone Mountain Audubon Sanctuary is a hidden jewel at the southern end of Maine's celebrated 100-Mile Wilderness, a greenway running along the Appalachian Trail corridor from Moosehead Lake to Baxter Park that the Appalachian Mountain Club and its partners are tirelessly working to protect. The sanctuary's 1,600 acres include rare old forest, sparkling ponds, exposed mountain peaks, and spectacular views.

Start the hike up Borestone via 0.8-mile Base Trail, which begins from the first kiosk on the shale-covered access road at the sanctuary's entrance gate. The trail begins steeply at first, though soon levels as it meanders up through

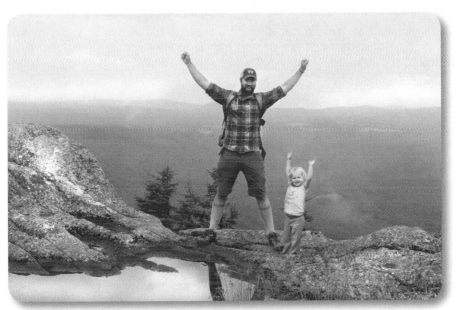

Father and daughter take a moment to celebrate their accomplishment at the summit of Borestone Mountain.

mature forest. Wildlife here is abundant: raccoons, owls, and woodpeckers nest in tree cavities; pine martens hunt for red squirrels; and goshawks fly overhead, searching for grouse. Base Trail intersects a gravel road at its terminus. Here, turn left to reach the Audubon Nature Center and Summit Trail.

The nature center—with interpretive displays and information about the area's natural and human history—is open most days between Memorial Day and Columbus Day, 9 A.M. to 4 P.M. Children will enjoy listening for bullfrogs or searching for leopard frogs and red-spotted newts on the shore of Sunrise Pond, just outside the center's doors. Picnic tables and benches surround the center. When hiking with young children, this may be the best turnaround spot. If you are seeking the summit, consider this scenic rest stop a fueling station for the strenuous climb ahead.

From the nature center, well-marked Summit Trail curves for 1.0 mile around the southern shore of Sunrise Pond. Poison ivy here can be abundant, and caution signs warn against going off-trail. The trail climbs steeply through spruce forest with the aid of more than 100 stone steps.

The final ascent to the West Peak is over exposed, green-blazed rock; keep the green triangles in sight to stay on-trail. Be prepared to use your whole body to climb in a few places, particularly where steel hand and footholds are provided. Though the views from the West Peak are impressive, hike an other 0.3 mile on exposed ledge toward the taller East Peak summit, at nearly

2,000 feet. Here, signage identifies many of the visible mountains, ponds, and streams within the impressive 360-degree panorama. Break out the binoculars and scan the shoreline below for moose—they've been known to frequent this area. Remember to keep your primary focus on the children, as the baldface summit does have steep ledges that kids should avoid. Retrace your steps down the mountain.

PLAN B: Don't plan a hike around Borestone without a visit to Little Wilson Falls, one of the highest waterfalls in Maine. (The "little" in its name refers not to the size of the waterfall but to the fact that it's on Little Wilson Stream.) It boasts multiple great swimming holes, scenic views of the gorge, and a main falls with a drop of more than 50 feet. From the sanctuary, turn right onto the unmarked dirt road immediately after crossing the bridge over Little Wilson Stream. Wherever this road branches, bear left. The road ends at a parking area next to Little Wilson Stream. A small set of falls is visible right from the parking lot, as is a great swimming hole. To access the larger falls, head upstream via a well-worn path that rises gradually for approximately 1.0 mile to the falls.

NEARBY: Cabins are available for rent within Borestone Mountain Audubon Sanctuary, between Midday and Sunset ponds. For more information and to make reservations, contact Maine Audubon. The town of Monson offers the closest restaurants and provisions.

Trip 23

All Ages $ 🚶 ✏ 🏊 🎩

Gorman Chairback Lodge & Cabins and Long Pond

Experience spectacular wilderness without compromising on comfort and amenities for the whole family.

Address: Off Katahdin Iron Works Road
Difficulty: Easy
Distance: Varies
Hours: 8 A.M.–9 P.M., seasonally
Fee: Gate fee at Hedgehog Checkpoint applies May–October ($7 for Maine residents ages 15–70, $12 for nonresidents ages 15-70; $10 for nonresidents ages 15–70 with printed reservation confirmations for Gorman Chairback Lodge & Cabins); free day-use access to Long Pond; contact Gorman Chairback Lodge & Cabins for lodging rates
Contact: Gorman Chairback Lodge & Cabins, 207-695-3085 (Greenville office), 603-466-2727 (reservations), outdoors.org/lodging/lodges/Gorman; North Maine Woods (Hedgehog Checkpoint), 207-435-6213, northmainewoods.org/ki-jo-mary/kijocheckpoints.html
Bathrooms: In the lodge and cabins
Water/Snacks: Meals, water, and snacks included with cabin stay
Maps: USGS Long Pond quad; *Maine Mountains Trail Map*, Map 2: F3 (AMC)
Directions by Car: From the traffic light in the center of Greenville, proceed north one block and turn right onto Pleasant Street. After 2.0 miles, the road becomes gravel. In 11.0 miles, stop, register, and pay the gate fee at the Hedgehog Checkpoint. Proceed 1.8 miles farther and turn right at the T intersection onto Katahdin Iron Works Road. Continue 3.5 miles and turn right onto Chairback Mountain Road. Continue for 1.3 miles and turn right onto the Gorman Chairback Lodge & Cabins driveway, which leads you directly to the facility and parking (45° 27.659′ N, 69° 19.014′ W). Note: Call ahead for winter driving directions. There is no fuel available in the area once you leave the state highways.

Appalachian Mountain Club's Gorman Chairback Lodge & Cabins is a wilderness destination offering unlimited hiking, skiing, and paddling opportunities within a 66,000-acre conservation and recreation area in the heart of Maine's

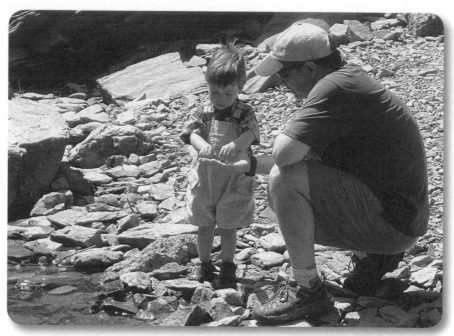

On the shores of Long Pond, father and son search for frogs, colorful rocks, and aquatic insects. (Photo courtesy of Anna Fincke)

rugged North Country. The hub is AMC's eco-friendly lodge, which has all the amenities a family could want: hot showers, restrooms, dining room, a wood-stove, comfy leather chairs, books and games, warm drinks, snacks galore, and a beautiful view of Long Pond and the mountains beyond. While day-use guests are welcome, this destination's remoteness calls for an extended visit. Eight private, cozy log cabins dot the picturesque shoreline, and cabin rental includes meals and unlimited access to canoes and trails.

In front of the lodge, a flotilla of canoes awaits, along with paddles and life vests for the whole family. This is excellent frog-catching territory, and the views are top-notch. The Barren-Chairback Range rises just beyond the pond while, to the north, the White Cap Range dominates the skyline. Rise early to try catching a glimpse of moose that occasionally visit the shoreline.

Launch from the dock and head out to explore. The clean, clear pond stretches for 3.0 miles, harbors native brook trout, and is dotted with several small islands for adventurous families to circumnavigate. Once on the water, head west, pass the second island, and hang a left. Directly behind the island is a half-moon cove with a lovely sandy beach on the left, a mere 0.5 mile from the dock. Here, you'll find picnic tables and calm waters, perfect for an afternoon swim.

PLAN B: Multiple trails of varying lengths and difficulties leave from the lodge. On-site staff members are happy to talk through which trails best suit your family's interests and abilities. Our favorite is 0.3-mile Hermit Point Nature Trail. Older kids can hike the trail themselves, feeling like independent adventurers as they trek through the woods and follow the curve of the inlet around to Hermit Point. Little do they know that their parents, sitting comfortably on Adirondack chairs in front of the lodge, can hear their every word and catch glimpses of them through the trees the whole time!

Kids will also love borrowing AMC nets and bug cages and heading out to see what critters wait in Henderson Brook. To access the brook, take the trail behind the bunkhouse, stay straight at the trail junction until it reaches the road, and follow the road to the culvert.

NEARBY: The closest large town is Greenville (20 miles away), where you will find ample provisions. Remember: there is no fuel available once you leave the state highways.

Trip 24

All Ages · $ · 🚶 · 🛶 · 🏊 · ⛺

Daicey Pond Campground

With nearby ponds and nature trails galore, this campground offers the perfect base camp for families exploring Baxter State Park.

Address: Daicey Pond, Millinocket
Difficulty: Easy
Distance: Varies
Hours: Seasonal
Fee: $14 summer entrance fee per vehicle for nonresidents; for cabin and campground fees, contact park
Contact: Baxter State Park, 207-723-5140, baxterstateparkauthority.com/camping/daiceypond.htm
Bathrooms: Outhouses are located throughout the campground
Water/Snacks: None
Maps: USGS Doubletop Mountain quad; *Maine Mountains Trail Map*, Map 1: E2 (AMC)
Directions by Car: From the intersection of ME 157/Central Street and Katahdin Avenue in Millinocket, proceed north on Katahdin Avenue and bear left at the Y intersection with Bates Street, staying on the main road. Bates Street shortly becomes Millinocket Road. Travel 16.0 miles to the Togue Pond Gatehouse, Baxter State Park's southern entrance. From the gatehouse, travel 10.0 miles to the sign for Daicey Pond. Turn left and drive another 1.5 miles to the campground parking area (45° 52.945′ N, 69° 1.907′ W).

Maine's wilderness is nearly synonymous with Baxter State Park: you can't rightly say you've explored the state's wild areas without a trip to this unique park. The 200,000-acre area encompassing its own mountain range, including Katahdin, was a gift to the people of Maine from Percival P. Baxter, former state governor. While the state's largest mountain is the park's jewel, drawing climbers from far afield who summit the 5,269-foot peak, there are myriad family-friendly areas to explore below treeline.

Daicey Pond Campground is an excellent home base for families visiting the park. The campground has ten rustic cabins of various sizes, all equipped with beds and mattresses, a woodstove, and gas lights. Picnic tables are

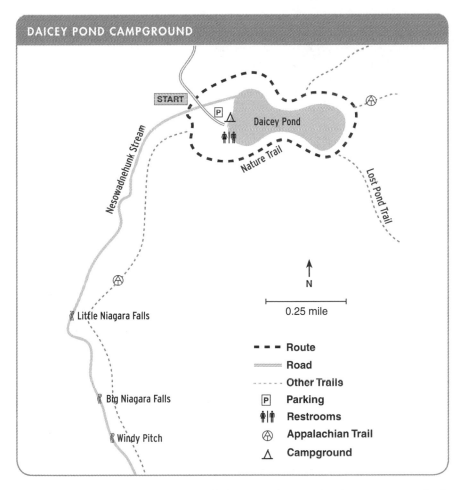

Route

Road

Other Trails

P   Parking

Restrooms

Ⓐ   Appalachian Trail

△   Campground

Nesowadnehunk Stream

START

Daicey Pond

Nature Trail

Lost Pond Trail

N

0.25 mile

Ⓐ

Little Niagara Falls

Big Niagara Falls

Windy Pitch

provided for outdoor cooking and dining. The pond-side campground offers great views and fishing opportunities, as well as hiking access to multiple
backcountry ponds and mountains. Canoes, paddles, and life jackets are available for rent. Children will delight in the kids' programs that take place here
most Saturdays throughout the summer. Activities range from tree bark rub-
bing to pond explorations with dip nets.

Favorite kid-friendly hikes originating from Daicey Pond Campground
include the 1.8-mile Daicey Pond Nature Trail. Flat terrain, plentiful wildlife,
and varied habitats make this a perfect adventure for even the smallest travelers. Start from the day-use parking area by heading out on the white-blazed
Appalachian Trail (AT) for 0.5 mile. Continue straight ahead on blue-blazed
Daicey Pond Nature Trail, leaving behind the AT as it veers right. As the hike
continues around the pond, numerous trail junctions present themselves, including those for three family-friendly trails, Grassy Pond Trail and Little and
Big Niagara Falls trails. Unless you're planning to venture out on one of the

adjoining trails, follow blue blazes to stay on Daicey Pond Nature Trail. Along the way, enjoy great views of Daicey Pond and the surrounding mountains, including Doubletop, Barren, Owl and, of course, Katahdin!

PLAN B: The best trails for families around Baxter's campgrounds tend to be nature trails. Kidney Pond Campground also offers rustic cabins and plenty of family-friendly activities. Great swimming holes within the park include South Branch Pond, Abol Pond, Matagamon Landing, and Ledge Falls, a natural waterslide north of Kidney Pond Campground.

NEARBY: Stock up on provisions in the town of Millinocket, 18 miles from the park's southern entrance.

GEAR UP

Encourage your budding naturalists by picking up a Naturalist Adventure Pack, available for free rental at Baxter State Park Visitor Center and all roadside ranger stations within the park. Pack contents include binoculars, guidebooks for identifying flora and fauna, dipping nets, and bug boxes.

Trip 25

All Ages · $ · 🐕 · 🚶 · 🛶 · ⛺

Shin Pond

Make the most of a trip to northern Maine by combining a fun, easy paddle with a rewarding hike to an unforgettable waterfall.

Address: 1489 Shin Pond Road, Mount Chase
Difficulty: Easy
Distance: Varies
Hours: No posted hours
Fee: Free for day use; contact Shin Pond Village for lodging and rental fees.
Contact: Shin Pond Village, 207-528-2900, shinpond.com
Bathrooms: At Shin Pond Village
Water/Snacks: Available at Shin Pond Village
Maps: USGS Shin Pond quad
Directions by Car: From I 95, Exit 264, take ME 11 north. In 19.8 miles, take a left onto ME 159/Shin Pond Road. Continue 10.0 miles to Shin Pond Village, a recreation resort. Rent kayaks and canoes at the main building or request permission to launch your own. To reach the launch, travel back on Shin Pond Road for 0.25 miles, turn right on Wapiti Road and immediately access the parking area on your right (46° 5.800′ N, 68° 34.115′ W).

Shin Pond Village is one of Maine's recreational gems, offering campsites, cottages, a general store and café, and canoe and kayak rentals, all in the heart of the wild North Country. Shin Pond itself offers great flatwater paddling opportunities, particularly on the lower pond. From the boat launch next to Shin Pond House, head west.

Lower Shin Pond spans approximately 3.0 miles long. Protected forests encompass the lake, and 2,440-foot Mount Chase rises gracefully to the south. Fall is the perfect time for a visit: the changing leaves show off their vibrant color as loons call on the lake and eagles perch in treetops above. Brook trout, bass, and salmon also call this pond home, so don't forget your pole!

PLAN B: For alternate paddling, head to the winding, marshy channel of the Sawtelle Deadwater, 10 miles northwest of Shin Pond Village on ME 159. Moose sightings here are often plentiful, particularly in the early mornings throughout May and June.

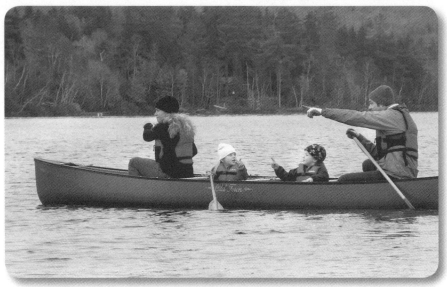

The calm waters of Shin Pond make this a great introductory paddle for families.

Take a short hike to the impressive Shin Brook Falls, one of Maine's most memorable waterfalls. From Shin Pond Village, travel northwest on Shin Falls Road for approximately 5 miles and follow signs on your left for Shin Falls. The trail begins to the right of the parking area and starts off through the woods on flat, easy terrain. When the trail forks at 0.1 mile, bear left and continue for another 0.3 mile to the upper falls. Keep small children close at hand as footing becomes more uneven. The trail ends at the upper section of the falls, where you can stare down at the cascading water below. This is your best, safest vantage point; the hike to the lower falls is too dangerous for children. Retrace your steps to the trailhead.

The northern entrance to Baxter State Park is 15 miles northwest of Shin Pond Village on ME 159 and offers an assortment of family-friendly recreational opportunities (see Trip 24).

NEARBY: The town of Patten is 10 miles southeast of Shin Pond Village and is home to the closest grocery store, as well as restaurants and cafés and the Patten Lumbermen's Museum, where you can learn all about Maine's logging history (lumbermensmuseum.org).

Northern
New Hampshire

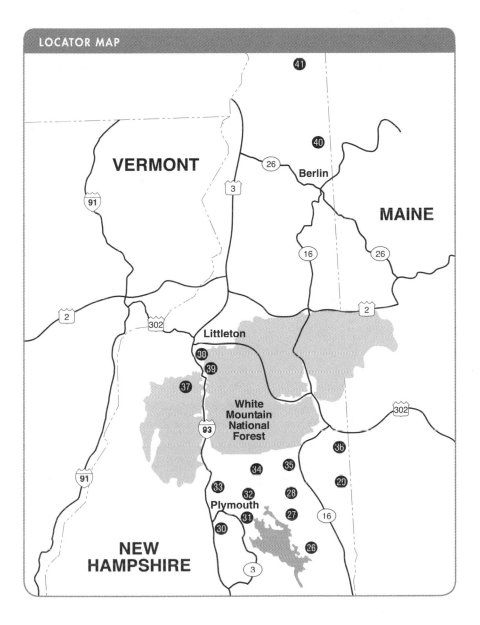

LOCATOR MAP

VERMONT

MAINE

Berlin

Littleton

White
Mountain
National
Forest

Plymouth

NEW
HAMPSHIRE

Trip 26

All Ages

Cotton Valley Rail Trail

A gem of a bike trip meets a paddle to a secluded island nature preserve. Enjoy plenty of wildlife viewing and a public beach, too!

Address: Depot Street (between Main Street and Glendon Street), Wolfeboro
Difficulty: Easy–Moderate
Distance: 3.8 miles, round-trip, to Albee Beach, 12.0 miles, round-trip, to Cotton Valley
Hours: No posted hours
Fee: Free
Contact: Wolfeboro Parks and Recreation, 603-569-5639, wolfeboronh.us/Pages/ WolfeboroNH_Recreation; Cotton Valley Rail Trail Club, cottonvalley.org
Bathrooms: At the railroad depot and at Albee Beach
Water/Snacks: At the railroad depot and at Albee Beach
Maps: USGS Wolfeboro quad
Directions by Car: From the intersection of NH 28 and NH 109 in Wolfeboro, continue west on NH 109 (Main Street). In 0.3 mile, turn right on Depot Street. Park anywhere along this street or farther down by the iconic red railroad depot (43° 35.156′ N, 71° 12.762′ W). If parking is full here, continue past the depot for additional overflow municipal parking lots.

The beautiful little town of Wolfeboro, its three lakes, its countless ponds, and its mountainous backdrop have attracted vacationers to its lakeshores for centuries. Biking the scenic Cotton Valley Rail Trail gives you the full Lakes Region experience as it takes you past (and sometimes across) Lake Winnipesaukee (the largest lake in New Hampshire), Back Bay (an inlet of Winnipesaukee), Crescent Lake, and 3,000-acre Lake Wentworth.

The 12-mile trail of packed stone dust has flat grades for the first 6 miles, but after Cotton Valley Rail Station it becomes much more rugged and undeveloped. Like most multiuse trails, Cotton Valley Rail Trail started out as a railway. In the 1990s it was turned into a trail for more universal use and is maintained by volunteers and the town, along with occasional grants from the state.

From the trailhead, the trail follows the shores of Back Bay. After pedaling over the Smith River, the trail reaches an intersection with NH 28 (Center

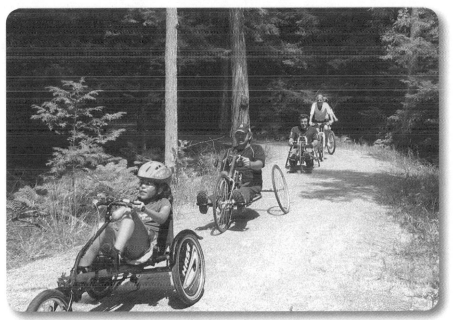

The gentle grades and firm surface of the Cotton Valley Rail Trail make it ideal for bikers of all ages and abilities. (Photo courtesy of Granite State Adaptive Sports)

Street), the busiest road crossing of the trip. The route continues on behind some residential areas and brings you to Mast Landing boat access on your right (see Plan B). Everyone will love what comes next: cycling across Crescent Lake on a narrow causeway with water on both sides of you! Over 100 years ago, engineers dumped hundreds of tons of granite into the water to create this narrow path so trains could cross on a straight course. If you like to fish, stop at one of the many pullouts or benches to try your hand at catching some sunfish, perch, or surprisingly large bass.

After reaching land, the trail crosses Whitten Neck Road. (Turn right on the road to see the low bridge over the Smith River where multiple generations of families continue the iconic summer tradition of jumping off next to the No Jumping sign; if you choose to join in, do so with care at your own risk.) Continue along the trail to a causeway crossing on Lake Wentworth. At 1.9 miles, the path winds through Albee Beach. Stop for a quick dip here if you choose, or save it for a treat on your way back.

Continue on the path over numerous small tributaries and a few road crossings to Fernald Station (3.0 miles) or the Cotton Valley Station (6.0 miles). These small brooks make for great exploration, and we have found many a great secret picnic spot along the grassy banks. Return the way you came.

PLAN B: Owned and managed by The Nature Conservancy and the Lake Wentworth Association, 100-acre Stamp Act Island is located on quiet Lake Wentworth, a favorite for paddlers and swimmers with only the occasional motorboat. To reach it from the intersection of NH 28 and NH 109 in Wolfeboro, head north on NH 28/109 for 1.2 miles to the Mast Landing boat put-in on Crescent Lake and parking area on your right (43° 35.604′ N, 71° 12.073′ W). Paddle along the left-hand (northeast) shore, paralleling the bike causeway to the narrow channel of the Smith River. While some small homes dot the shoreline, this is a peaceful section of the trip, complete with good swimming and jumping opportunities at a small bridge. After 0.6 mile, you will emerge on Lake Wentworth.

Head east through a small cluster of islands with homes, to the much larger, uninhabited Stamp Act Island beyond them (2.0 miles). Circumnavigate the island to reach a small picnic beach on its west end (4.2 miles). Aside from this designated picnic beach, the island is closed to human exploration so that the birds and animals can exist in peace; please respect the creatures here. If you are lucky, you may see herons and even some nesting bald eagles. Return back to Mast Landing through the Smith River channel (6.2 miles).

NEARBY: Wolfeboro is home to many excellent ice cream shops in the lively downtown Main Street, and there are numerous sandwich shops, pizza parlors, and high-end waterfront eateries as well. In fall, head to Devylders Farm on Pleasant Valley Road for apple picking, hayrides, doughnuts, a farm stand, and pumpkins. Canoes and kayaks are available to rent through outfitters in many towns around neighboring Lake Winnipesaukee.

Trip 27

Ages 8+

Mount Roberts and Fall of Song

A little-known mountain range offers this trail to a summit with open ledgy views over Lake Winnipesaukee.

Address: 455 Ossipee Park Road, Moultonborough
Difficulty: Moderate
Distance: 4.8 miles, round-trip
Hours: No posted hours for trails; contact Castle in the Clouds for facility hours and season
Fee: Free
Contact: Lakes Region Conservation Trust, 603-253-3301, lrct.org; Castle in the Clouds, 603-476-5900, castleintheclouds.org
Bathrooms: At Castle in the Clouds
Water/Snacks: Castle in the Clouds offers a full service café and a hot dog and ice cream stand located next to Shannon Pond
Maps: USGS Melvin Village and Tamworth quads; *Castle in the Clouds Conservation Area Hiking Trails Map*, 2e (Lakes Region Conservation Trust, 2014), lrct.org/explorelearn/maps-guides
Directions by Car: From the intersection of NH 25 and NH 109, head east on NH 109 to the intersection with NH 171. Veer left here onto NH 171 and continue for 0.5 mile. Turn left onto Ossipee Park Road. Follow Ossipee Park Road for 1.3 miles to the trailhead parking area in front of the gate to Castle in the Clouds (43° 43.913′ N, 71° 19.496′ W), which is directly across the road from the entrance to a spring water bottling plant. You can also take the very scenic drive to Castle in the Clouds directly from NH 171, 2.2 miles from its intersection with NH 109; a fee to use this road will be charged at the gate.

Featuring open ledgy ridges, waterfalls, and vistas of Lake Winnipesaukee and the White Mountains, the Ossipee Mountains are sparsely populated and provide a great wilderness experience for hikers. The majority of the property in the Ossipee Range is owned and managed by the Lakes Region Conservation Trust, which offers excellent maps of the area and runs programs year-round. The trailhead itself is on the property of Castle in the Clouds, a historic estate now part of the Castle in the Clouds Conservation Area. Mount Roberts is perhaps the most attractive of the mountains in this range, as it offers moderate grades and excellent views for much of the trip up the ridge. While many

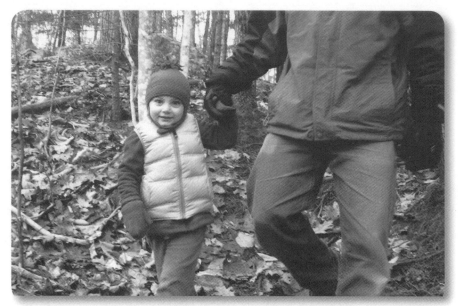

Fall is a great time to hike in the Castle in the Clouds
Conservation Area—just be sure to bundle up!

New England hikes require hours of slogging through dense forest to reach an open summit, Mount Roberts's exposed ridges give you wide-open skies and vistas from about halfway up to the summit.

From the trailhead parking, walk up the road through the gate onto the Castle in the Clouds property. Follow the road for a couple hundred yards until you see Shannon Pond ahead. This pond is a great place to catch frogs or feed the immense brook trout raised here.

Turn left at the intersection and head up the hill toward the horse stables. No trip to Mount Roberts is complete without a stop here to see the horses on your way up or down. Trail rides are also available; find more information at ridingintheclouds.com.

Continuing past the stables, follow the signs for Mount Roberts Trail, which leaves to the right. The trail winds up Roberts Ridge through the woods and soon rewards you with numerous open ledges with commanding views of Lake Winnipesaukee and the Belknap Range to the south. As you climb higher, the trail continues through sections of open ridge and thick fir forests reminiscent of Narnia or Middle-earth. Let your imagination run wild as you walk through these quiet and magical hollows. Continue on through the woods to the open summit with views of the Sandwich and Presidential ranges to north.

After a picnic or snack at the top, head back down the way you came for a 4.8-mile round-trip.

PLAN B: The excellent Brook Walk Trail leads to a series of five waterfalls, including the idyllic Fall of Song. While there are no mountain views, this shorter hike (1.6 miles, round-trip) will delight all ages as it descends along the banks of a babbling brook and cascading falls. From Shannon Pond, walk across the dam and head right on Brook Walk Trail. Cross a bridge over the brook. Stay left along the banks of Shannon Brook as you pass Bridal Veil Falls, Roaring Falls, Twin Falls, and Whittier Falls, and finally reach the 40-foot Fall of Song. To return, hike back up the way you came.

NEARBY: NH 25 in Moultonborough offers a fine collection of restaurants and delis. A special treat is the Old Country Store, the oldest store in America, which has operated since 1781. More than just a tourist stop, it offers old-fashioned candies, cheddar cheese, iron goods, and picnic fixings.

WHY IS THE OSSIPEE MOUNTAIN RANGE CIRCULAR?
The Ossipee Mountains are one of the world's best examples of a ring dike. During the Jurassic Period, circular cracks formed in the surface of the earth and were filled by molten lava coming up from below, forming a circle of new, igneous rock. Look at a topographic map or satellite images of the Ossipee Mountains to see their almost perfectly circular shape.

Trip 28

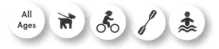

All Ages

Bearcamp River

A peaceful mountain valley paddle, complete with fun riffles, deep swimming holes, and a trout-stocked river that is navigable most of summer.

Address: Whittier Road (between NH 113/Tamworth Road and NH 25/Bearcamp Highway), Tamworth
Difficulty: Easy
Distance: 4.75–5.25 miles
Hours: No posted hours
Fee: Free
Contact: n/a
Bathrooms: None
Water/Snacks: None
Maps: USGS Tamworth and Ossipee Lake quad
Directions by Car: *NH 25 put-in/take-out*: From the intersection of NH 16 and NH 25 in Ossipee, head west on NH 25. After 100 yards or so, a bridge crossing over the Bearcamp River and the canoe/kayak put-in are on your right (43° 49.151′ N, 71° 12.331′ W). Park a car here to establish a shuttle for option #1. Alternatively, this is the put-in for option #2. *Whittier Road put-in:* From the NH 25 put-in/take-out, continue over the bridge and continue for 0.9 mile to Whittier Road (Old NH 25). Turn right and proceed 1.7 miles to a grassy spot on the right past the white house on the right and the red barn on the left. While using the put-in, park temporarily near mailbox 514 (43° 49.886′ N, 71° 15.282′ W); a small trail leads through the woods to the river. *Do not leave a car here while you paddle.* Park farther west on Whittier Road (Old NH 25) at the convenience store about 0.75 mile upriver, or park at the NH 25 take-out and plan to bike back to this put-in. *Ossipee Lake take-out:* For option #2 the best take-out option is at the end of Nichols Road off of NH 16. From the intersection of NH 16 and NH 25, head south on NH 16 for 1.75 miles and turn left on Nichols Road. Follow Nichols Road for 1.0 mile until it ends at Ossipee Lake (43° 48.407′ N, 71° 9.850′ W).

This tranquil river trip combines perfect conditions for lazily paddling through a beautiful mountain valley, and swims and picnics at sandy beaches along the way. The river is stocked with trout, and we've seen many large ones here. This section is fairly untamed: not too many houses are in sight, and you will

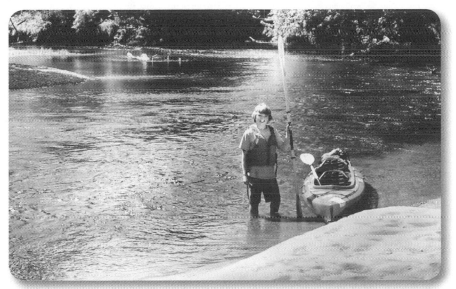

Sandy beaches and a slow current make the Bearcamp River a relaxing and pleasant paddle.

have to watch out for "strainers" (trees that have blown down into the river) particularly when the water is high in spring or after prolonged heavy rainfall. You can paddle a shorter trip from Whittier Road to NH 25 (option #1), a longer paddle traveling from NH 25 to Ossipee Lake (option #2), or make a full day of it by combining the trips.

Consider establishing a bike shuttle for the whole family to travel the 2.6 miles between the NH 25 take-out and the Whittier Road put-in. We've found that this is often our kids' favorite part of the day! Option #2 is far friendlier for car shuttles or for adults and older kids who are comfortable biking across a busy state highway. Combining the two would require a car shuttle or a longer bike ride.

Option #1 Whittier Road to NH 25 (4.75 miles)

The river is shallowest for the first 500 yards; when we paddled it in June, we had to drag the boat over a couple of scratchy sections. The rest of river is navigable for most of summer and many deep pools make for excellent swimming on a hot day.

The paddle is remarkably sunny, dappled with shade as you pass through the red maple and pine floodplain forest along the way. Half the fun of this paddling trip is stopping at the beaches and coves along the way. Kids get a Robinson Crusoe-like thrill when they hop off the boat on an unexplored beach for a picnic, and you'll spend hours playing in the clean river sand, searching for treasures washed up in the last flood. Please be courteous of posted private property.

After winding past many beaches and pools, pass under a covered bridge (3.75 miles) and arrive at the take-out at NH 25 (4.75 miles). If you're adding Option #2 to your day, continue under the bridge.

Option #2: NH 25 to Ossipee Lake (5.25 miles)

The first couple miles from the NH 25 bridge are punctuated by numerous campgrounds and cottages, but the paddling is tranquil and there are many more fine beaches and swimming holes to enjoy. Past the NH 16 bridge (3.0 miles) the river's character becomes a bit more secluded, and there are some good picnic beaches along the winding bends. At the mouth of the river in Ossipee Lake, a popular rope swing on the right attracts paddlers and boaters for summer fun.

When the river empties into the lake, turn left and follow the shore past some tightly spaced cottages and a small cove; a sandy beach and the terminus of Nichols Road are 0.7 mile from the end of the river (5.25 miles).

PLAN B: The Remick Country Doctor Museum and Farm (remickmuseum.org) in Tamworth is a real treat and the farm animals will entrance the kids. Also in Tamworth is the Lyceum, a unique combination mercantile, café, and education center; they have many weekend naturalist programs for kids and adults.

NEARBY: Tamworth (intersection of NH 113 and NH 113A) has a small collection of interesting local businesses, a café, and restaurants, as well as a vibrant Saturday farmers' market. The intersection of NH 25 and NH 16 in Ossipee is your closest bet for convenient and quick food on your way south or north. Canoe and kayak rentals are available at outfitters in nearby Conway.

Trip 29

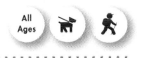

Foss Mountain

A very short, gentle walk to a bald granite knob reveals open vistas of the White Mountains and acres and acres of blueberries!

Address: Foss Mountain Road (between Stewart Road and Willis Bean Road), Eaton
Difficulty: Easy
Distance: 0.5 mile, round-trip
Hours: No posted hours
Fee: Free
Contact: Eaton Conservation Commission, 603-447-2840, eatonnh.org
Bathrooms: None
Water/Snacks: None
Maps: USGS Conway quad
Directions by Car: From the intersection of NH 25 and NH 16 in Ossipee, head east on NH 25 for 5.3 miles. Turn left on NH 153 and head north for 10.0 miles, passing King Pine Ski Area on your left. Eventually you will pass Crystal Lake on your right. At the northern end of the lake, turn right on Brownfield Road. In 1.0 mile, turn right on Stewart Road. Continue for 1.0 mile, then turn right on Foss Mountain Road, and proceed for 1.5 miles to the small trailhead parking area on your left (43° 52.927′ N, 71° 2.205′ W) with blueberry fields on your right.

Foss Mountain is the perfect hike for toddlers ready to hit the trail on their own two feet, for older kids who want to pick blueberries, or anyone looking for a great view with little effort. Put simply, Foss Mountain has it all: a gentle walk, astounding views for a mountain this small, and acres upon acres of blueberries which are ripe for the picking June through August. You will not be disappointed.

From the parking area, cross the road and proceed through the gate. The trail winds its way through blueberry fields right from the beginning. These fields are commercially harvested, so please do not stop and pick berries here—there are plenty of wild blueberries at the summit.

After a few hundred feet the trail ascends gently up into the woods, passes through another few hundred yards of woods, and emerges onto a 33-acre

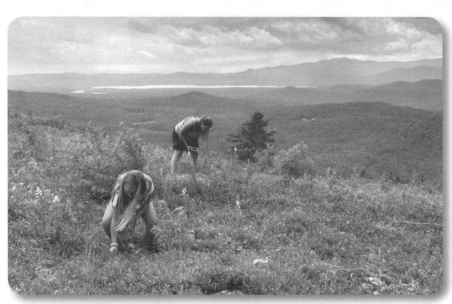

Picking blueberries on the open summit of Foss Mountain, you may feel transported to a page from Blueberries for Sal.

granite knob lushly carpeted with wild blueberry bushes as far as you can see. At the information kiosk, turn right to hike the last few dozen yards to the summit. As you pick your way slowly up to the summit, you can imagine yourselves as characters in *Blueberries for Sal*, except hopefully you won't surprise any bears!

At the summit (0.25 mile), expansive views in all directions make it seem as if you are on top of the world, even though the peak is only 1,647 feet high. Ossipee Lake spreads out below the mountain to the south, and Mount Chocorua in the Sandwich Range, Mount Washington in the Presidential Range, and Mount Shaw in the Ossipee Range are all clearly visible. Spread out for a sunny picnic and fill up on blueberries for dessert. When it's time to go, just head back the way you came.

PLAN B: The Foss Mountain Alpaca Farm on Foss Mountain Road is definitely worth a stop. The owners raise alpacas and ragdoll cats, and they welcome visitors to come see and pet the animals. White Lake State Park on NH 16 has an excellent public beach, perfect for an after-hike swim.

NEARBY: Stop in for picnic supplies on NH 153 in Eaton before your hike up Foss Mountain. The bacon in our BLTs from the Easton Village Store was still hot when we arrived at the summit! Nearby Conway also has a wide variety of pubs and restaurants.

OPEN SUMMITS

Why are some summits open and why are some forested? At high eleva-tions above treeline, many summits are open because the conditions are too harsh, windy, and cold for trees to grow to a significant height, or at all. Foss Mountain's summit isn't above treeline, but it was originally kept open by fires caused by lightning. Now, humans help nature maintain this special place. Volunteers with weed-whackers keep the saplings down so that the blueberries can thrive here, and the Eaton Conservation Commission even brings in what it calls a Brontosaurus (an excavator with a giant grinding wheel on it that takes down trees of any size) to help keep the ground open and clear to create ideal berry habitat.

Want to go on a real-life treasure hunt, running through the woods to gather clues and win a race? Or do you want to use GPS units and advanced maps to locate hidden objects in the woods? Then grab your gear and try out orienteering and geocaching! Many families take part in these activities while they're hiking, biking, or paddling—or even when they're getting to know a new city. You may need a few new skills to get going, but your family will be even more prepared in the outdoors once you've mastered the basics.

Orienteering: This sport calls on your navigational skills (typically using a map and compass) to find "control points" (which are usually markers permanently attached to a tree or rock). Orienteering was originally developed as a military training exercise, but the thrill of using maps to find your way helped it become very popular as a recreational activity. On orienteering courses, control points are laid out over the landscape within a set area, but you'll use detailed maps rather than established trails to find your way to each one. Your ultimate goal is to locate the control points in the correct order and to return to the starting point with your best possible time. Many people simply walk the course and find it challenging enough to find each control point using just their wits, a map, and a compass. More advanced participants do the course while at a full-tilt run!

Our families have done orienteering courses all over the country—from Arizona to Washington to New Hampshire. Sewall Woods in Wolfeboro, New Hampshire, has a family-friendly, introductory-level course; maps and instructions are available online so you can give it a shot on your own. More information and maps for the Sewall Woods course are available at the Up North Orienteers Club website, upnoor.org. General information on the sport is available at orienteeringusa.org.

Geocaching: If you prefer your navigation skills bolstered by something battery-powered, give geocaching a go. You'll use a GPS-enabled device to find "caches" (hidden objects) that are spread out over a very large area—a park, an entire town, city, or even a state. Participants log on to one of many geocaching websites and get GPS coordinates for caches nearby. Caches are often hidden in plastic containers or ammo boxes to protect them from the elements, and once participants find the object, they either mark a log at the site or enter their accomplishments online. The beauty of geocaching is that it gets people outside to locations they may have never visited and is very thrilling for kids (and adults) when they search high and low and finally find the hidden cache! For more information and to get involved, see geocaching.com.

Trip 30

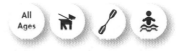

Pemigewasset River

As the Pemigewasset River meanders through a pastoral valley, its gentle current and fun riffles carry you to sandy islands that beckon to be explored.

Address: 37 Green Street, Plymouth
Difficulty: Easy
Distance: 6.0-mile paddle to Bridgewater, one-way; 12.75-mile paddle to New Hampton, one-way
Hours: No posted hours
Fee: Free
Contact: New Hampshire Department of Environmental Services, Rivers Management Protection Program, 603-271-2959, des.nh.gov/organization/divisions/water/wmb/rivers
Bathrooms: None
Water/Snacks: None
Maps: USGS Plymouth and Holderness quads
Directions by Car: *To the put-in in Plymouth (Green Street):* From I-93, take Exit 27 for NH 175. Head west on NH 175A across the large bridge over the Pemigewasset River. Make an immediate left after the bridge onto Green Street. Head south for 0.25 mile past Plymouth District Court to the river access point immediately on the left (43° 45.436′ N, 71° 41.194′ W). There is a large sign for "Pemigewasset River Car Top Boat Access" with plenty of parking. *To the take-out in Bridgewater (River Road):* From the intersection of I-93 and NH 104, head west on NH 104 for 1.4 miles over the bridge to River Road. Turn right on River Road and head north for 6.0 miles to the pullout on your right. (43° 40.965′ N, 71° 39.146′ W). *To the take-out in New Hampton (NH 104):* From the intersection of I-93 and NH 104, head west on NH 104 for 1.2 miles over the bridge to the large gravel parking lot and put-in on the right (43° 36.423′ N, 71° 39.855′ W).

The paddle described here is all quick-moving flat water; there are no rapids, but the current will carry your boat along a peaceful ride through a beautiful valley and a couple of fun riffles along the way. Combined with plenty of swimming, island exploring, and world-class picnicking, this is a great trip for a sunny summer afternoon. The fishing is good (plenty of brook trout, rainbow trout, and smallmouth bass patrol these waters) and for extra fun on hot

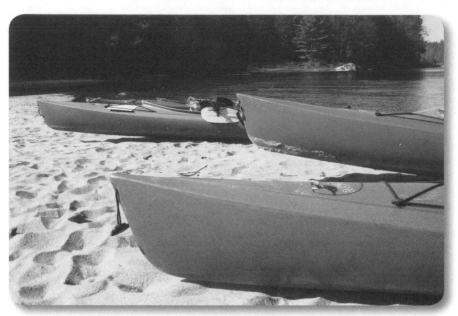

The Pemigewasset River is lined with sandy islands that are ideal for sunning, resting, and picnicking.

days, bring along an inner tube or two that the kids can ride and you can tow behind the boat.

The Pemigewasset River drains a large swath of the southern White Mountains and winds gradually through the Pemigewasset Valley until it joins the Winnipesaukee River to become the Merrimack River. If you were to follow the Merrimack south through New Hampshire and Massachusetts, you would eventually drift out into the Atlantic near Plum Island, Massachusetts.

From the boat put-in in Plymouth, you will meander along the sandy-bottomed river, past many great swimming opportunities. You will pass a few sandy beaches and then a golf course on your left. Even though many towns are nestled in the Pemigewasset Valley and a state highway and an interstate cross it, you will rarely see much evidence of mankind from the river. Instead, you'll be able to enjoy the sounds of the river, the birds singing, and the wind rustling through the trees.

Stop at one of the many sandy islands for lunch and a siesta, and then continue on toward your preferred take-out: either the one in Bridgewater (6.0 miles) or the one in New Hampton (12.75 miles). If you're traveling all the way to New Hampton, be aware: the current slows down in the last couple miles due to a dam downstream of the take-out, so you will need to save up energy for some paddling at the end. The full trip will take 3–5 hours, depending on how many breaks you take along the way.

PLAN B: On a rainy day, consider visiting the Squam Lake Science Center (nhnature.org, 603-968-7194) in nearby Holderness, which includes excellent exhibits on New Hampshire natural history, nature walks, lake cruises, and even some zoo-type wildlife exhibits—including a mountain lion and bears!

In better weather, the nearby Baker River in Plymouth has many easy access points for tubing and paddling. The busy but amazing Lost River Gorge (lostrivergorge.com, 603-745-8031) is located at the headwaters of the Pemigewasset River on NH 112 in North Woodstock. This deep, narrow gorge features plenty of caves to explore and is sure to delight everyone.

NEARBY: Plymouth has a fine collection of food options, ranging from Thai to country Italian to excellent delis and pubs. Biederman's Deli serves giant sandwiches and has a foosball table that will please all ages; call ahead to order boxed lunches to-go for your island picnic. Canoe and kayak rentals are also available at outfitters in Plymouth.

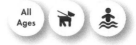

West Rattlesnake Mountain and Five Finger Point

A well-worn path leads to exhilarating open vistas of Squam Lake, with an option to continue on to crystal clear swimming and jumping rocks!

Address: NH 113 (between Metcalf Road and Pinehurst Road), Sandwich
Difficulty: Easy–Moderate
Distance: 1.8 miles, round-trip, to West Rattlesnake Mountain; 5.3 miles, round-trip, to Five Finger Point
Hours: No posted hours
Fee: Free
Contact: Squam Lakes Association, 603-968-7336, squamlakes.org
Bathrooms: None
Water/Snacks: None
Maps: USGS Squam Mountains quad; *AMC White Mountain National Forest Map & Guide*, L6 (AMC); squamlakes.org/map
Directions by Car: From the intersection of I-93 and NH 25 in Ashland, head east on NH 25 through Ashland. Continue for 3.7 miles to Holderness and turn left onto NH 113. Continue for 5.5 miles to the gravel trailhead parking area on your right (43° 47.356′ N, 71° 32.906′ W).

West Rattlesnake Mountain is well loved for a reason: the truly easy, beautiful, 0.9-mile hike and its expansive vistas south over Squam Lake and the Belknap Mountains are rewarding. A sunny Saturday in summer may not be a solitary experience here, but the simple beauty of this natural oasis of rocky ledges and wide-open skies will still be enjoyable. The flat ledges at the summit make a perfect picnic spot, and there are plenty of nooks and crannies to find a private spot to enjoy the view. The path is short and its grades are gentle, making this a perfect trip for the smallest hikers. And if you're up for a longer day, you can continue on to Five Finger Point for beaches, swimming, and world-class jumping into the crystal clear waters of Squam Lake.

From the trailhead, head south on Old Bridle Path. Climbing gently through deciduous forest of maple and birch, this trail has been beautifully maintained and contains many fine examples of rock staircases and water bars.

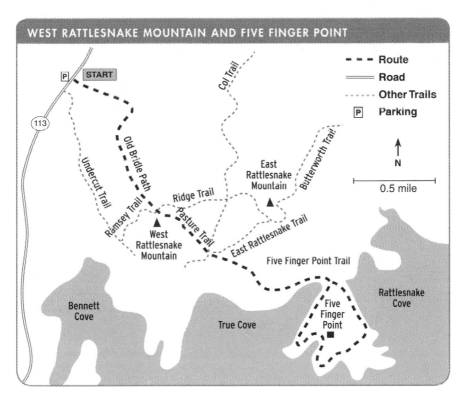

Route
Road
Other Trails
P   Parking

N

0.5 mile

Col Trail

START
P

113

Old Bridle Path

Undercut Trail

Ramsey Trail

Ridge Trail

Pasture Trail

West
Rattlesnake
Mountain

East
Rattlesnake
Mountain

Butterworth Trail

East Rattlesnake Trail

Five Finger Point Trail

Bennett
Cove

True Cove

Five
Finger
Point

Rattlesnake
Cove

With over 25,000 users a year, the volunteers of the Squam Lakes Association maintain this trail for heavy use and to control erosion. You, too, can get involved in their trail building efforts or make a donation to help with upkeep at the trailhead.

After a very gentle 0.9-mile ascent, you will start to get glimpses of open sky and finally reach the open ledges of the summit. The islands and lush shoreline of Squam Lake spread before you, and you may feel as if you are at the helm of a giant granite ship!

After picnicking at the summit, head back the way you came for a 1.8-mile round-trip, or continue on to Five Finger Point for a full 5.3-mile adventure.

From the summit of West Rattlesnake Mountain, find the intersection for Pasture Trail and follow toward the lake. After a 0.4-mile descent, stay left on East Rattlesnake/Five Finger Trail. In 25 yards, continue on Five Finger Trail as it branches off to your right. Follow this downhill for another 0.7 mile to the start of the 1.3-mile Five Finger Loop which follows the contours of a peninsula with five distinct fingers of land, with picturesque bays and inlets in between. Here you'll encounter a remarkable virgin, old-growth beech-oak-pine forest; these trees are noticeably larger than any of the other trees in the area. Many beaches and jumping rocks dot the shoreline, so leave time to play on a hot day. Return the way you came, up and over West Rattlesnake and down the Old Bridle Path to the trailhead, for a 5.3-mile round-trip.

PLAN B: The Sandwich area is full of fun outdoor activities and exploration. On a rainy day, consider visiting the Squam Lake Science Center (nhnature. org, 603-968-7194) in nearby Holderness, which includes excellent exhibits on New Hampshire natural history, nature walks, lake cruises, and even some zoo-type wildlife exhibits—including a mountain lion and bears!

NEARBY: Both Holderness and Sandwich have great collections of pubs, restaurants, and cafés. For an iconic Sandwich experience, visit the out-of-the-way and legendary Sandwich Creamery (134 Hannah Road, Sandwich) for ice cream, cheeses, and a visit with farm animals. A *New Hampshire Atlas and Gazetteer* (DeLorme) is recommended for finding your way on these winding back roads!

Trip 32

Ages 8+ 🐕 🚶 🏊 ⛺

Mount Israel

A ledgy, open summit with great views of the Sandwich Range. The magical Beede Falls nearby offer hours of swimming, sliding, and stream exploration.

Address: Diamond Ledge Road, Sandwich
Difficulty: Challenging
Distance: 4.2 miles, round-trip
Hours: No posted hours
Fee: Free for day use; contact the Mead Conservation Center for camping fees
Contact: White Mountain National Forest, 603-536-6100, www.fs.usda.gov/main/whitemountain; Mead Conservation Center, 603-968-7336, squamlakes.org/recreation/mead-conservation-center
Bathrooms: None
Water/Snacks: None
Maps: USGS Center Sandwich quad; *AMC White Mountain National Forest Map & Guide*, L7–K7 (AMC)
Directions by Car: From the intersection of NH 113 and NH 109, head west on NH 113 for 0.1 mile and veer right onto Grove Street. After 0.4 mile, continue straight onto Diamond Ledge Road and follow this for 1.9 miles where Diamond Ledge merges with Sandwich Notch Road. After 0.2 mile, Diamond Ledge Road branches off again to the right; follow it for 0.3 mile where the road ends at a small parking lot in front of a farmhouse (43° 49.717′ N, 71° 29.038′ W).

This hidden gem of a hike starts at the Mead Conservation Center, operated by the Squam Lakes Association. Wentworth Trail is 4.2 miles out-and-back and is moderately steep, but the rewards at the top are sure to brighten the spirits of your youngest hikers. This trip can be done in a day, but also makes an ideal camping destination. Camp at the Mead Conservation Center campsites at the trailhead (visit the center's website to make reservations) and spend a whole day on Mount Israel, and another day at Beede Falls. Everything is within walking distance of your campsite!

Wentworth Trail up Mount Israel ascends to the left of the white farmhouse at the trailhead and climbs steadily until you reach a stream (0.8 mile). After the stream crossing, the trail continues to climb steadily, offering a couple of

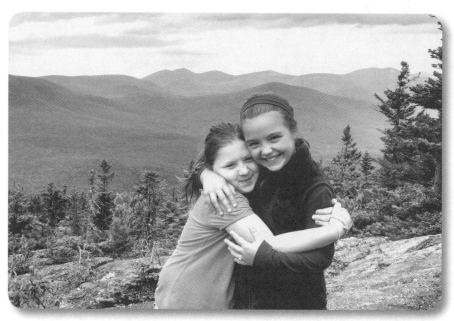

Friends celebrate reaching the summit of Mount Israel.

level spots along the way to take breathers. This trail has been well maintained in recent years and you will find many finely constructed rock staircases on your way up. At 1.5 miles, the trail passes some nice ledge views to the south (on your left); this is a great turnaround spot for a short day. At 2.0 miles, the path reaches the long summit ridge with partially obstructed views to the north. Continue along the rolling summit to Mead Trail. Veer right here; 150 feet beyond the intersection, the trail emerges onto the true summit (2.1 miles) with excellent views of the entire Sandwich Range and to the peaks of Waterville Valley in the north. The open ledges are perfect for a picnic lunch and maybe a siesta on a nice sunny day. Descend the way you came up (4.2 miles).

From the Mead Conservation Center, Beede Falls are just a 15-minute walk (0.5 mile on flat ground) or a short drive away. If walking, head west on Bearcamp River Trail from the trailhead (a right turn if you're coming down from Mount Israel). Pass the Mead Conservation Center campsites and continue on past the underhanging Cow Caves, which make for fun exploration. Soon the sound of Beede Falls greets you. Your family will likely want to spend hours exploring. The main fall features an overhanging drop that you can walk behind, or stand under the falls themselves if the flow is not too strong. Young children will love the 50-foot-wide sandy pool (1–4 feet deep). No jumping here as it is too shallow!

We have spent hours exploring the small pools and slides above and below the main fall. On a sunny day, these fine ledges would be perfect for lounging on a towel and soaking in the rays as you swim and slide the hours away.

PLAN B: On your way to or from the conservation center, don't miss the giant-sized table and chairs randomly placed in a farm field along the road. Standing at least 15 feet tall, they are a truly bizarre sight! (On Mount Israel Road, just off Diamond Ledge Road.) Nearby Rattlesnake Ledge and Five Finger Point trails offer great views of Squam Lake and excellent swimming and jumping opportunities.

On a rainy day, consider visiting the Squam Lake Science Center (nhnature.org, 603-968-7194) in nearby Holderness, which includes excellent exhibits on New Hampshire natural history, nature walks, lake cruises, and even some zoo-type wildlife exhibits—including a mountain lion and bears!

NEARBY: Sandwich has a great collection of pubs, restaurants, and cafés. For an iconic Sandwich experience, visit the out-of-the-way and legendary Sandwich Creamery (134 Hannah Road, Sandwich) for ice cream, cheeses, and a visit with farm animals. A *New Hampshire Atlas and Gazetteer* (DeLorme) is recommended for finding your way on these winding back roads!

Trip 33

Ages 5+ · $ · 🐕 · 🚶

Welch Mountain and Dickey Mountain

This perfect, ledgy loop hike up and over two small mountains leads to amazing views of Franconia Ridge, Waterville Valley, and the Pemigewasset Valley.

Address: Orris Road (between Gateway Road and Harris Road), Thornton
Difficulty: Moderate
Distance: 4.5 miles, round-trip
Hours: No posted hours
Fee: $3 per vehicle
Contact: White Mountain National Forest, 603-536-6100,
    www.fs.usda.gov/whitemountain
Bathrooms: Pit toilet
Water/Snacks: None
Maps: USGS Waterville Valley quad; *AMC White Mountain National Forest Map & Guide*, K5 (AMC)
Directions by Car: From I-93, take Exit 28 for NH 49 and go east for about 6.0 miles. Turn left, cross a bridge and follow upper Mad River Road 0.7 mile. At Orris Road turn right and go 0.6 mile to the parking area on the right (43° 54.234′ N, 71° 35.335′ W).

This popular hike over Welch and Dickey mountains is perhaps one of the most beautiful and satisfying trips in New England, with everything you could ask for: a mostly gentle grade (with some exciting slabs to climb near the top), excellent views from the ridge, two summits, and the satisfaction of a loop hike! While it may be challenging for the toddlers (although it's totally possible with an occasional ride from mom or dad), kids age 6 and up will love this hike for the wide-open skies and amazing granite slabs. In bad weather and wet conditions, be cautious on this hike: the slabs can be very slippery and the ridgeline is exposed.

Starting at the trailhead, go right on Welch-Dickey Loop Trail to start a counterclockwise loop. The hike up Welch Mountain is steep in spots and it is much easier and safer to hike up these sections than descend them. Stroll up gradually through the birch and maple forest along a pleasant babbling brook.

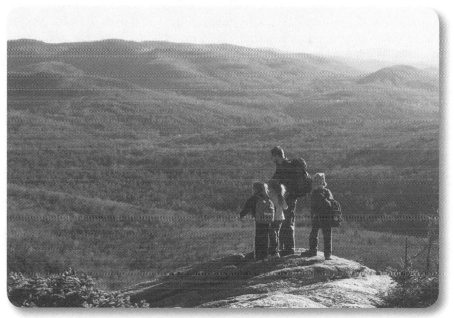

*The granite knobs and open slabs of Welch and Dickey mountains
provide expansive views of the surrounding ranges.*

Soon the trail will begin to climb, and at about the 1.3-mile mark you will come to the first open ledges with views to the south and the Mad River below.

For the next couple miles you will be largely out in the open on granite ledges, ridges, and summits. Continue on up the open slabs to the left. Travelling on granite slabs can be fun and scenic, but keep the toddlers close as a tumble here could have serious consequences. In wet conditions, this section is not recommended. However, in dry weather, the hiking could not be better, with sure footing beneath you and open skies above.

These mountains are known for their open ledges and rock outcroppings, but at one time, this whole area was covered in a thick forest of white pine and oak trees. But these prominent peaks are a target for lightning, and a massive lightning fire in the 1880s and harsh weather conditions denuded the summit. Additional lightning strikes since then have kept the summits and ridge open. Today, patches of blueberries thrive on these craggy ledges from June through August, so be sure to leave time to explore off-trail for these sweet treasures. (Read more about open summits in Trip 29.)

Soon you will come to the open summit of Welch Mountain. There are plenty of great picnic spots and views here: Mount Moosilauke to the northwest; Waterville Valley and Mount Tecumseh to the east; and the Franconia Ridge to the north. You will see the knobby summit of Dickey Mountain just to the north, with a short descent and a quick climb to reach the summit there.

Continuing on counterclockwise from Dickey, descend over the large granite dome with a steep drop on your left—keep the kids close here. Soon you'll be back into the woods for the last mile of the loop.

PLAN B: You could spend a full day exploring the multiple unnamed swimming and fishing spots along the Mad River that parallels NH 49 up into Waterville Valley. One excellent nearby swimming spot, "The Eddie," *is* named and can be located at a Forest Service pull-off on NH 49, 2.3 miles west of the turn-off on Mad River Road for the Welch-Dickey trailhead.

NEARBY: Great dining options abound in this area. A few good taverns, restaurants, and ice cream stands can be found in Campton near the intersection of NH 49 and NH 175, and nearby Ashland has very good options as well.

Trip 34

Cascade Brook

Perfect on a hot summer day, this pleasant walk cuts through the woods to a string of some of the state's finest swimming holes.

Address: Boulder Path Road (between W Branch Road and Cascade Ridge Road), Waterville Valley
Difficulty: Easy
Distance: 3.1–3.6 miles, round-trip
Hours: No posted hours
Fee: Free for day use; contact Snow's Mountain Chairlift for current lift ticket pricing
Contact: White Mountain National Forest, 603-536-6100, www.fs.usda.gov/whitemountain; Snow's Mountain Chairlift, 603-236-4807, waterville.com/summer-play-explore/summer-snows-chairlift.html
Bathrooms: None
Water/Snacks: None
Maps: USGS Waterville Valley quad; *AMC White Mountain National Forest Map & Guide*, J6 (AMC); map available May–October at the base of the chairlift
Directions by Car: From I-93, Exit 28 for NH 49, go east 11.2 miles. Once you are in the village of Waterville Valley, stay to the right, passing the school on your right and a small pond and some hotels on your left. Turn right at the golf course onto Boulder Path Road and continue for 0.4 mile. Just past the tennis courts, you will see the buildings of Waterville Valley Academy on your right and a large parking lot (43° 57.576′ N, 71° 30.511′ W); park here.

There are many brooks named Cascade Brook in New Hampshire, but on a hot summer day, this is the best one. This short hike leads to a string of swimming holes and rock waterslides. Plan for plenty of time to relax and swim—you won't want to leave!

The first and best option to reach Upper Snows Mountain Trail and the pools (described in detail here) is to simply hike up the abandoned ski trails of Snow's Mountain. These trails are sunny, wide open, and dotted with blueberries. While the ski area has been closed for decades, the chairlift here runs June through October, bringing mountain bikers and hikers up to the top. You can ride the lift instead to take 1.0 mile off the round-trip hike.

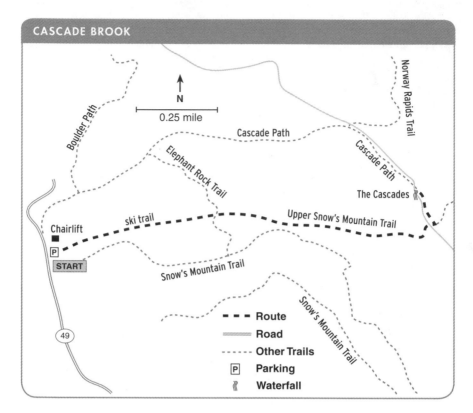

CASCADE BROOK

N
0.25 mile

Boulder Path

Cascade Path

Norway Rapids Trail

Elephant Rock Trail

Cascade Path

The Cascades

ski trail

Upper Snow's Mountain Trail

Chairlift

P

START

Snow's Mountain Trail

Snow's Mountain Trail

49

- - - Route
═══ Road
- - - - Other Trails
P   Parking
≀   Waterfall

From the parking lot, stay right and walk up your choice of the abandoned ski trails—they all lead to the top of the ski lift (0.5 mile). To the right of the bottom of the lift is Phil's Hill Training Center, an artificial ski slope used year-round by Olympic and X-Games athletes to practice massive aerial flips and twists.

Continue up the ski trails, picking blueberries along the way if you're visiting between June and August. At the top of the lift there are a couple of picnic tables that make a great rest stop. Head right into the woods on Upper Snows Mountain Trail, which is actually an abandoned woods road that gradually descends to Cascade Brook. Mountain bikers also use this trail, so keep an ear out for bikes behind you. After 0.8 mile, this pleasant and wide trail arrives at a bridge over Cascade Brook. Take a left immediately before the bridge onto Cascade Brook Trail.

After a couple hundred yards, you will come to the first of many swimming holes on your right (1.6 miles). The first swimming hole is our favorite, with perfect jumping spots from 2 to 6 feet above the water's surface. The water is crystal clear and emerald tinted, and feels just like paradise on a hot summer day. Stick your head under the cascade for a backcountry shower, or if you time your trip to arrive midday, sun yourself on the rock slabs (the slabs are shady the rest of the day).

Continue on down Cascade Brook Trail for at least three other swimming holes within the next 0.25 mile, all with good jumping, slabs, and even some rock slides for the adventurous. Reaching some of them will require crossing the brook and finding the best path down. You can spend hours here in a Tom Sawyer and Huck Finn state of mind, swimming, sunning, jumping, and relaxing. If you are ever able to pull yourself away, just return the way you came.

PLAN B: Hunt down your very own secret fishing and swimming spots. Just drive along NH 49 from Waterville Valley along the Mad River and park at one of the many gravel pull-offs and start exploring your way up or down the river.

Waterville Valley has become a mountain biking destination, with many of the trails accessible from the Snow's Mountain Chairlift (for a fee), or just grab a map at the base of the lift and head out for free on the National Forest Trails. Multiple campgrounds in the area make this an ideal multiday trip.

NEARBY: Great dining options abound in this area. Waterville Valley has many restaurants, ice cream shops, and a pizza parlor. A few good taverns, restaurants, and ice cream stands can be found in Campton near the intersection of NH 49 and NH 175, and nearby Ashland has very good options as well.

Trip 35

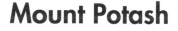

Ages 8+

Mount Potash

Just off of the iconic Kancamagus Highway, this small-yet-mighty mountain features open ledges with spectacular views, a gentle grade, and a quiet, secluded trail.

Address: NH 112 (across from Passaconaway Campground), Albany
Difficulty: Moderate
Distance: 4.4 miles, round-trip
Hours: No posted hours
Fee: Free
Contact: White Mountain National Forest, 603-536-6100,
    www.fs.usda.gov/whitemountain
Bathrooms: At trailhead, maintained Memorial Day to Columbus Day
Water/Snacks: None
Maps: USGS Mount Tripyramid quad; *AMC White Mountain National Forest Map & Guide*, J8 (AMC)
Directions by Car: From the intersection of NH 16 and NH 112 in Albany, head west on NH 112 (Kancamagus Highway) for 14.2 miles to the Downes Brook–UNH–Mount Potash trailhead on the left (43° 59.652′ N, 71° 22.159′ W), directly across the road from the Passaconaway Campground.

Mount Potash is a delightful hike for families: short, gradual, and highly rewarding with open ledges providing excellent views in all directions. Even the drive up the Kancamagus Highway is an experience. Travelers from all corners of the world flock to this famous road for its serpentine curves up the Swift River and excellent views of the White Mountains. While this area can get crowded on sunny weekend days, you can escape the masses on Mount Potash and enter the calm silence of the North Country woods.

From the parking lot, head out on Downes Brook Trail for 0.3 mile to the intersection with Mount Potash Trail and make a right. Climb gently through the woods to a crossing of Downes Brook, which may be difficult in spring or following heavy rains. The trail crosses a logging road and climbs past evidence of logging activity on your right.

After passing through a beautiful hemlock forest, the trail climbs more steeply over the forest floor, which has been worn down to bedrock and is

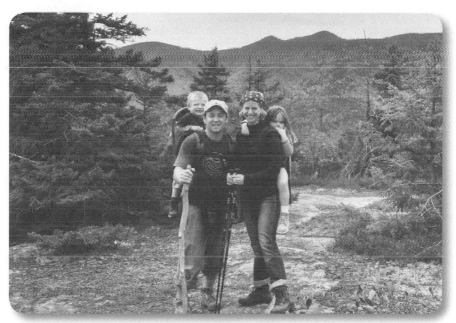
Young families on outdoor adventures will inevitably carry their children for many miles in baby backpacks—but it is all worth it when you reach a beautiful view!

laced with tree roots. Climb these roots like a ladder as you ascend toward the ridge. Soon sunlight pokes through the trees and scattered ledges offer limited views toward Mount Passaconaway. The trail ascends steep granite ledges to the wide-open summit itself (2.2 miles).

At the summit, your reward is expansive views in all directions and plenty of great spots to picnic. To the east, look for Mount Passaconaway and Hedgehog Mountain; directly to the west is a mountain with the best name of any we've heard: the Fool Killer. Look to the north to see Crawford Notch and the Presidential Range. Return the way you came.

PLAN B: Swimming holes abound on the Swift River that parallels NH 112, with some popular ones like Lower Falls attracting hundreds of visitors on a hot sunny day. For a less busy swim after your hike, head to Jigger Johnson Campground, park, and hike down to the Swift River near campsite 60 or 49.

NEARBY: Conway and North Conway have excellent dining options, including Thai, Indian, pizza, burgers, and well-renowned breweries, as well as ice cream stands.

Food can be the highlight of any outdoor trip, not just something we eat to stay alive! Food provides energy, sustenance, and happiness on the trail, so plan good meals to make trips with kids happy and fun.

For day trips, pack a good picnic lunch and *always* bring along some on-the-go treats that will provide quick energy to keep folks moving, such as trail mix, dried fruit, or fresh fruit. When you reach that steep section of trail and the young legs are giving out, the heat is oppressive, and the bugs are biting, busting out a hidden chocolate bar could make the difference between hiking on to your destination happily or turning back early! Food can be the ultimate motivator.

For multiday trips, plan out and pack your meals ahead of time. Providing balanced nutrition is important, as you will be spending lots of energy hiking, swimming, biking, and paddling! A grid-style menu ensures you have every meal accounted for and can also be used as a shopping list. Yours could look something like this:

	THURSDAY	FRIDAY	SATURDAY	SUNDAY
BREAK-FAST	On the road—stop for bagels	Pan fried bagels, cream cheese, fruit, coffee	Bacon and eggs, toast, fruit, coffee	Sticky buns in the Dutch oven, fruit, coffee
LUNCH	Salami, cheese, crackers, pickles, trail mix	PBJ, fruit, trail mix	Salami, cheese, crackers, pickles, dried fruit, cookies	On the road—stop in for pizza
DINNER	Campfire burgers, baked potatoes, coleslaw, cookies	Dutch oven mac and cheese, hot dogs, fruit	Quesadillas, fruit, Dutch oven pineapple upside down cake	Home!

For multiday trips, bring a day or two's worth of extra food. Weather, injuries, and other emergencies can keep you out longer than you'd intended, so bring along some extra pasta and cheese to make survival grub. Or you may just go through more food than you'd planned. Extra hot meals come in handy when kids—especially the 10-and-up crowd—arrive in camp starving after a long day of hiking or paddling or when it is raining and cold and you're all in need of a bit more to eat. Our favorite 5-minute hot snack on a rainy day is backcountry pad thai: cook up a packet of ramen noodles, dump the water after it's cooked, add the seasoning packet to taste, along with a healthy tablespoon or so of peanut butter (and all the hot sauce you like) for a 5-minute backcountry gourmet delight!

Trip 36

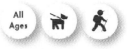

Black Cap

A great first hike for little ones, Black Cap offers fantastic views on open ledges with just a mile-long climb.

Address: Hurricane Mountain Road (between Timberland Drive and Green Hill Road), North Conway
Difficulty: Easy
Distance: 2.5 miles, round-trip
Hours: No posted hours
Fee: Free
Contact: Conway Conservation Commission, 603-447-3811, conwaynh.org/boards/conservation; The Nature Conservancy, 603-356-8833, nature.org/newhampshire
Bathrooms: None
Water/Snacks: None
Maps: USGS North Conway East quad; *AMC White Mountain National Forest Map & Guide*, I12 (AMC)
Directions by Car: From the intersection of NH 16 and NH 112 in Conway, head 0.8 mile north on NH 16. Just past the intersection with NH 153, turn left and continue north on NH 16. After 7.4 miles, turn right on Hurricane Mountain Road (closed to vehicles November through mid-May). Proceed 3.7 miles to the signed trailhead on the right (44° 4.095′ N, 71° 4.312′ W).

Black Cap is perfect for the smallest hikers or for those short on time who want to have great views with little effort. It is a local favorite and you are sure to see others on the trail for their daily run or walk. The summit is large and open, so even on a busy Saturday, you should be able to find a quiet spot with a great view to enjoy a picnic lunch.

From the parking lot, head up wide-and-rooty Black Cap Trail through Conway Common Lands State Forest and The Nature Conservancy's Green Hills Preserve. Hiking in this area has been popular for more than 100 years, but the ridgeline between Black Cap, Peaked Mountain, and Middle Mountain was permanently protected in 1990. The Nature Conservancy now manages more than 4,200 acres of land here, forming a continuous tract of open space adjacent to the state forest and the White Mountain National Forest.

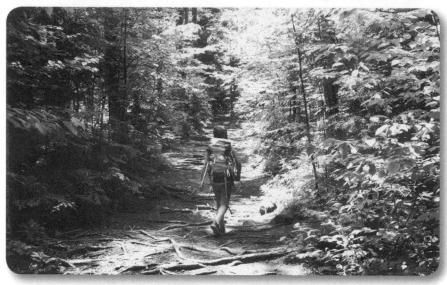

Navigating the exposed roots on paths like Black Cap Trail can be tricky!

The trail continues on a moderate uphill grade. Stay left at both Cranmore Trail (0.7 mile) and Black Cap Connector (0.8 mile). Continue 0.3 mile to open ledges and the bald summit (1.1 miles). Forest fires cleared the summit of all vegetation at the turn of the twentieth century, so you can now enjoy excellent views in all directions. Stop here for a picnic, but bring your bug spray in June and early July; the blackflies can drive the kids (and you) crazy!

Continue south beyond the summit to Black Cap Connector Trail (1.3 miles). Turn right here and continue, backtracking below the summit, to the northern intersection with Black Cap Trail (1.7 miles). Turn left on Black Cap Trail, and head back to the parking lot (2.5 miles).

PLAN B: Stop at the Mount Washington Observatory Weather Discovery Center (mountwashington.org/education/center) to learn about the extreme weather in the White Mountains. Swim in the cascading pools at nearby Diana's Baths (44° 4.480′ N, 71° 9.812′ W) on a hot day. Head up Cathedral Ledge Road in Echo Lake State Park to the famed Cathedral Ledge for views back across the Mount Washington Valley. Or hike the steep, fun, rock-staircase trails from the parking area to the base of the 700-foot-tall cliffs to watch the rock climbers.

NEARBY: You are sure to find a restaurant that suits any taste in North Conway, from barbecue to Thai and Indian, to locally sourced flatbread pizzas.

Trip 37

Long Pond

Nestled in the foothills of the Kinsman Range, this high-country pond offers hours of island exploring, wildlife viewing, and fishing.

Address: Long Pond Access Road, Benton
Difficulty: Easy
Distance: 2.0 miles, round-trip
Hours: No posted hours
Fee: Free
Contact: White Mountain National Forest, 603-536-6100, www.fs.usda.gov/whitemountain
Bathrooms: None
Water/Snacks: None
Maps: USGS East Haverhill quad; *AMC White Mountain National Forest Map & Guide*, H2–I2 (AMC)
Directions by Car: From I-93, take Exit 32 and head west on NH 112, which joins NH 116 in about 11.0 miles. After another mile, continue left on NH 116, crossing the Wild Ammonoosuc River, and continuing for 1.6 miles. Turn left on Long Pond Road. After 2.5 miles, turn right onto Long Pond Access Road, and follow signs for the picnic area and parking (44° 3.517´ N, 71° 52.629´ W).

A paddle on Long Pond is like a trip deep into the wilderness. The shoreline is completely undeveloped, and its unspoiled islands and the surrounding Kinsman Range make it an exhilarating and special destination. Early morning on the pond is often misty and calm, with the best chances of viewing wildlife like otters, beavers, deer, and moose. Afternoons are warmer, but the wind can pick up and make the water choppier. Early evening is always a pleasant time; the winds usually calm down so you can enjoy a peaceful sunset and maybe even catch a massive brook trout. And it's hard to beat a sunset picnic on an island.

The northern end of the lake near the put-in is dotted with islands that have the potential for great adventure. For a young child, there are few things more exciting than pretending you're an intrepid explorer, or you're making a fort for shelter against unseen forces, or that you're a castaway and have to survive in this wild place.

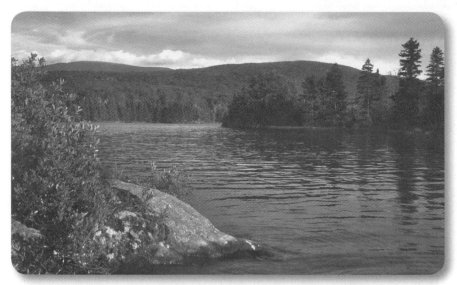
Long Pond offers majestic views of Mount Moosilauke to the east, and the blueberry picking is top-notch! (Photo courtesy of Andrew Rebeiro)

Many marshy coves and bays offer interesting exploring and excellent wildlife viewing. Maple, birch, and spruce dominate the forest here. On the southern end of the pond there are a couple of rocky points where you can land your boat. Spend an hour or a day surveying the nooks and crannies of this crystal clear pond.

Dispersed camping is available in the White Mountain National Forest, but no overnight parking is allowed at the pond itself.

PLAN B: Explore the captivating waterfalls and swim in the potholes of Agassiz Basin on NH 112. To get there from Long Pond, head back to the intersection of NH 116 and NH 112. Turn right on NH 112 and proceed 10.1 miles to a small white building on the right with a gravel parking lot (44° 1.733′ N, 71° 43.084′ W). Find other excellent swimming holes at the other gravel pull-offs along NH 112 heading toward North Woodstock. The Lost River Gorge (see Trip 30) is also nearby.

NEARBY: The sister towns of Lincoln and North Woodstock have dozens of restaurants, with enough options to please just about anyone. Several of the eateries in downtown North Woodstock are just steps away from the very pleasant Cascade Park (44° 1.927′ N, 71° 41.192′ W), which features wading pools and rock slides for a pre- or post-dinner swim! Canoe and kayak rentals are available at outfitters in Lincoln.

Trip 38

Ages 5+ | $ | 🐕 | 🥾 | 🏊

The Falls on Basin–Cascades Trail

The excitement of discovering multiple swimming holes and backcountry cascades will be the highlight of this trip—bring your swimsuit!

Address: The Basin, Franconia Notch Parkway (I-93), Lincoln
Difficulty: Moderate
Distance: 2.0 miles, round-trip
Hours: No posted hours
Fee: $3 White Mountain National Forest parking pass, payable at trailhead
Contact: White Mountain National Forest, 603-536-6100,
    www.fs.usda.gov/whitemountain
Bathrooms: At the trailhead
Water/Snacks: Water available at the trailhead
Maps: USGS Lincoln and Franconia quads; *AMC White Mountain National Forest Map & Guide*, H4 (AMC)
Directions by Car: From I-93, take the exit for the Basin, 2.2 miles north of Exit 34A on the northbound side or 3.6 miles south of Exit 34B on the southbound side. Park in the trailhead parking lot (Northbound: 44° 7.161′ N, 71° 40.883′ W; Southbound: 44° 7.417′ N, 71° 40.957′ W). If you park in the lot on the northbound side of the interstate, follow signs for the Basin to the pedestrian way beneath the road (0.2 mile).

This has to be one of the Hipple family's favorite day trips in all of New Hampshire. The highlights include multiple backcountry swimming holes and waterfalls, fishing for brook trout, and the chance to visit the Appalachian Mountain Club's Lonesome Lake Hut (see Plan B). This type of trip is best experienced on a hot summer day, when the humidity and heat force us out of our homes and up into the mountains. Depending on your family's ambition and energy level, you can turn around at any one of the many falls to make your trip either shorter or longer.

The Basin brings hundreds of visitors a day to view its water-carved granite potholes. Don't let the size of the crowds scare you away though: very few of them venture beyond the first 0.2 mile of asphalt trail. After admiring this busy and beautiful spot, make a left on Basin-Cascades Trail. Soon the fumes of the tour buses and the voices of the crowds will fade into the distance as the

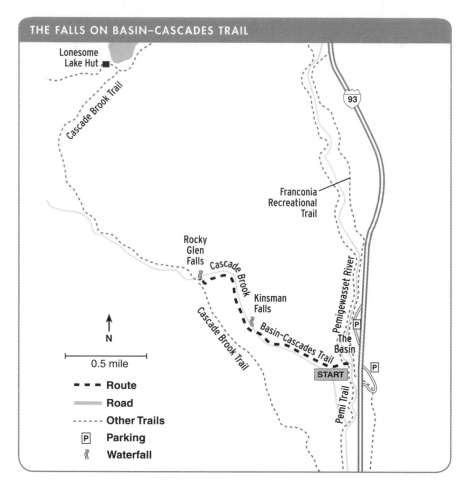

THE FALLS ON BASIN–CASCADES TRAIL

Lonesome
Lake Hut

Cascade Brook Trail

93

Franconia
Recreational
Trail

Rocky
Glen
Falls

Cascade Brook

Kinsman
Falls

Cascade Brook Trail

Basin-Cascades Trail

Pemigewasset River

P

The
Basin

START

P

N

0.5 mile

Pemi Trail

- - - Route
=== Road
- - - - Other Trails
P   Parking
⌇   Waterfall

songs of the birds and the babbling Cascade Brook take over. The contrast is immediate and almost startling.

The trail climbs up the north bank of the Cascade Brook with some interesting unnamed slab slides and drops spread out along the first 0.25 mile. Kinsman Falls (0.4 mile) is the first named falls on the trail, and this 15-foot plunge into a deep, swimmable pool begs to be explored.

Moving up the trail you will cross the brook and pass multiple unnamed cascades and swimming spots. We counted ten swimmable holes in between Kinsman Falls and Rocky Glen Falls, but there are probably more. See how many you can find! Many of these have small gravel beaches and shallow sections perfect for toddlers to while away the hours, and some open slabs make excellent sunning and picnic spots. On one particularly hot day, we simply traveled up this trail in our swimsuits and sturdy sandals, hopping from one swimming hole to the next.

Finally, you will reach Rocky Glen Falls (0.9 mile), an idyllic and semi-hidden gem that is our favorite of the hike. The water drops 35 feet through a narrow gorge into a small pool at the bottom. But the best part of Rocky Glen is hidden at the top. Continue on up the trail until you come to the point where the trail crosses the brook. Walk down the brook carefully to reach the top section of Rocky Glen Falls and you will find an excellent swimming hole that is so deep we couldn't find the bottom! Making your way down to the pool is tricky, but the best way we found was to cross over to the north side of the brook (opposite the trail) and descend a small path to some jumping spots as well as a spot where you can ease in from shore. If Rocky Glen Falls is your final destination, turn around here for a 2.0-mile round-trip.

PLAN B: To continue on to the magical Lonesome Lake Hut, continue on Basin-Cascades Trail across the brook where it intersects with Cascade Brook Trail. Turn left here and continue up gradually through birch and maple forests for 1.6 miles to the shores of the high-country Lonesome Lake. Excellent views of Cannon Mountain across the lake await, and if you've come this far, continue another 0.2 mile to AMC's Lonesome Lake Hut, a backcountry lodge where hikers are free to stop in and get a cup of tea, some fresh baked goods, and shelter from the weather. You can even make arrangements to spend the night here, complete with dinner and breakfast; for more information, visit outdoors.org/lodging. Turn around at the hut and head back to the parking lot for a 5.2-mile round-trip.

NEARBY: The sister towns of Lincoln and North Woodstock have dozens of restaurants and will be able to please just about anyone.

Trip 39

Franconia Notch Recreation Path

With gentle grades, swimming options, and amazing scenery in one of New Hampshire's most dramatic locations, this bike trip has everything you need for the perfect day.

Address: Flume Gorge and Visitor Center, 852 Daniel Webster Highway (US 3), Lincoln
Difficulty: Easy–Moderate
Distance: Up to 17.6 miles, round-trip, biking; many shorter options available
Hours: No posted hours
Fee: Free
Contact: 603-745-8391, nhstateparks.org/explore/state-parks/flume-gorge.aspx
Bathrooms: At the Flume, the Basin, and Lafayette Place Campground
Water/Snacks: At the Flume, the Basin, and Lafayette Place Campground
Maps: USGS Lincoln and Franconia quads; *AMC White Mountain National Forest Map & Guide*, G4–H4 (AMC)
Directions by Car: *To the Flume Gorge and Visitor Center:* From I-93, take Exit 34A and continue on NH 3 and follow signs to the Flume (1.0 mile southbound; 0.5 mile northbound). Proceed to the north end of the parking lot (44° 5.824′ N, 71° 40.878′ W) to reach the bike path. *To the Skookumchuck Brook Trailhead:* If you choose to bike the entirety of the trail in one direction, leave one vehicle at the Skookumchuck Brook Trailhead, which is the bike path's northern terminus. From the Flume, follow US 3 north for 0.4 mile until it merges with I-93. Follow I-93 for 6.9 miles up and over Franconia Notch to Exit 35 for US 3 Daniel Webster Highway. Follow US 3 for 0.6 mile to the trailhead parking on the right (44° 12.200′ N, 71° 40.859′ W).

There are few places in New Hampshire or even New England that can match the scenic vistas found in Franconia Notch. This bike ride, which can range from just a few miles to a full 17.6-mile day, lets you see this gorgeous area from the seat of your bike. It is recommended for experienced bike riders ages 6 and up, or any age at all in a bike trailer or child carrier. While much of it is gradual, there are a few short, steep sections that may be a safety concern for kids who are inexperienced with properly braking while descending. Younger children

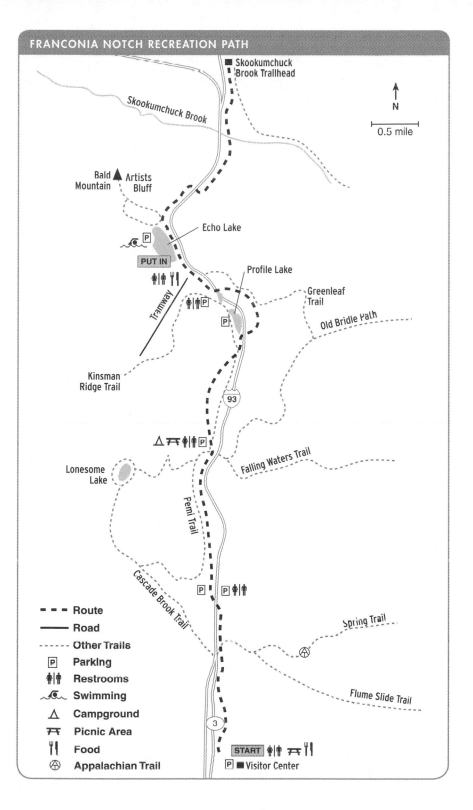

Skookumchuck
Brook Trailhead

N

0.5 mile

Skookumchuck Brook

Bald Mountain
Artists Bluff

Echo Lake

P

PUT IN

Profile Lake

Greenleaf Trail

Old Bridle Path

Tramway

P

Kinsman Ridge Trail

93

Falling Waters Trail

Lonesome Lake

Peni Trail

Cascade Brook Trail

Spring Trail

Flume Slide Trail

- - - Route
——— Road
- - - Other Trails
P Parking
Restrooms
Swimming
△ Campground
Picnic Area
Food
Ⓐ Appalachian Trail

3

START

P ■ Visitor Center

can safely walk down the steeper sections with adult supervision. Helmets are always recommended.

Depending on the ability of your group or how much time and energy you have, choose any of the following destinations as a turnaround point to create the perfect trip itinerary.

The Basin (1.8 miles)

By starting your ride at the Flume Gorge, you can pedal your way up the hill and coast home at the end of your ride. Head out of the parking lot on the paved trail, which is perfect for bikes of all types. Stay to the right if you are riding slowly so others can pass you.

In 1.8 miles the trail reaches the Basin, a unique and beautiful geologic formation in the Pemigewasset River featuring granite potholes and swirling clear water. If you'd like to explore the area and escape the crowds, refer to Trip 38 for a 0.5-mile side trip to Kinsman Falls.

Lafayette Campground (3.5 miles)

This beautiful 1.7-mile section of the trail follows the Pemigewasset River closely. Many brook trout have been caught in these waters, so bring along a collapsible rod to try your hand. Lafayette Campground is a hub of activity for summer day-hiking in the area. It is a major gateway to AMC's High Huts, including Lonesome Lake Hut (see Trip 38, Plan B) and Greenleaf Hut, and you may see some scruffy hut "croo" members carrying loads of food and supplies up to the High Huts for dinner.

Profile Lake (5.5 miles)

This 2-mile section has many rolling hills and veers farther away from I-93. When coming down, be sure to stay on the brakes.

As you head north from the campground, look for the beaver dam on your right. The path passes under the Cannon Cliffs (former home of the Old Man of the Mountain) and skirts Profile Lake's northwestern shore.

Skookumchuck Brook Trailhead (8.8 miles)

This 3.3-mile section goes up and over the notch. From Profile Lake, ride north past the former Old Man viewing area, past Echo Lake, and beneath the ski area at Cannon Mountain. Just past Echo Lake, you will pass NH 118. For a great view of the notch, park the bikes just to the west on US 118 and scamper up Artists Bluff, a popular and beautiful walk.

Proceeding north, the path takes a beautiful, gradual descent to the Skookumchuck Brook Trailhead on US 3.

PLAN B: The Flume has amazing wooden boardwalks that suspend you over the raging waters and falls. There is an admission fee, but it is a fun place to visit nonetheless. The Flume Scavenger Hunt, available online, is especially enjoyable. See nhstateparks.org/explore/state-parks/flume-gorge.aspx for more details.

And for a cold dip after your long bike ride, explore the Moosilauke Brook's fun potholes along the side of the road on Lost River Road (NH 112). From the intersection of NH 112 and US 3 in North Woodstock, head west on NH 112 for approximately 1.5 miles. Choose a dirt pull-off on the left and start exploring!

NEARBY: The sister towns of Lincoln and North Woodstock have dozens of restaurants and will be able to please just about anyone.

THE OLD MAN OF THE MOUNTAIN

Forever enshrined on New Hampshire's state seal, license plates, road signs, and even the state quarter, the Old Man of the Mountain was a unique geologic formation on the Cannon Cliffs in Franconia Notch that resembled an old man's face if viewed from just the right angle. Beloved by generations of locals and visitors, the cliffs sadly collapsed in May 2003, due to gravity and natural damage from ice that formed in the cracks in the cliffs.

Since the 1920s the state park system and a local volunteer family, the Nielsens, had noticed the expanding cracks in the cliff and worked to preserve the cliffs and minimize the damage caused by ice and water. They used a mix of chains, cables, and concrete to keep the cliff together, but eventually the twin forces of water and gravity proved to be too much to battle.

Lovers of New Hampshire the world over mourned the loss of this symbol that represented the craggy, individualist, and tough nature of the state's people. The symbolism of this rocky profile was perhaps best summarized hundreds of years ago by the famous statesman and New Hampshire native Daniel Webster: "Men hang out their signs indicative of their respective trades; shoemakers hang out a gigantic shoe, jewelers a monster watch, and the dentist hangs out a gold tooth; but up in the Mountains of New Hampshire, God Almighty has hung out a sign to show that there He makes men."

Trip 40

All Ages 🐾 🛶 🏊 ⛺

Lake Umbagog

Lake Umbagog is a North Country treasure, teeming with wildlife, surrounded by boreal forests, and dotted with islands and beautiful backcountry campsites.

Address: Umbagog Lake State Park, NH 26 (between Mountain Pond Road and La Fleur Avenue), Cambridge
Distance: 2.0–24.0 miles, round-trip
Difficulty: Easy–Challenging
Hours: No posted hours
Fee: Free for day use, fee for camping and for canoe or kayak rentals
Contact: Lake Umbagog State Park, 603-482-7795, nhstateparks.org/explore/state-parks/umbagog-lake-state-park.aspx; Umbagog National Wildlife Refuge, 603-482-3415, www.fws.gov/northeast/lakeumbagog/index.html
Bathrooms: At campground
Water/Snacks: At campground
Maps: USGS Umbagog Lake South and Umbagog Lake North quads; nhstateparks.org
Directions by Car: From the intersection of NH 16 and NH 26 in Errol, head east on NH 26 for 7.3 miles to Lake Umbagog State Park. Proceed through the campground to the boat put-in and parking area on the left (44° 41.927′ N, 71° 3.067′ W).

Lake Umbagog (pronounced um-BAY-gog) is a place of immense beauty, solitude, and wilderness. Home to the largest concentration of nesting loons and ospreys in New Hampshire, it is also home to copious numbers of moose, bears, lynxes, coyotes, minks, and bobcats. It sprawls over 7,538 acres in a remote corner of northern New Hampshire, making it logistically difficult to reach, and therefore quiet and peaceful for those who do visit. The relatively shallow lake (average depth is 15 feet) is the second largest in the state and is chock-full of warm- and cold-water fish. Bass, landlocked salmon, brook trout, and perch are prolific here, and it is rare for a fishing trip to go by without at least one catch-of-the-day dinner. On one trip we caught a giant lake trout, saw an eagle soaring overhead, and found a moose in a secluded cove—*all within five minutes.*

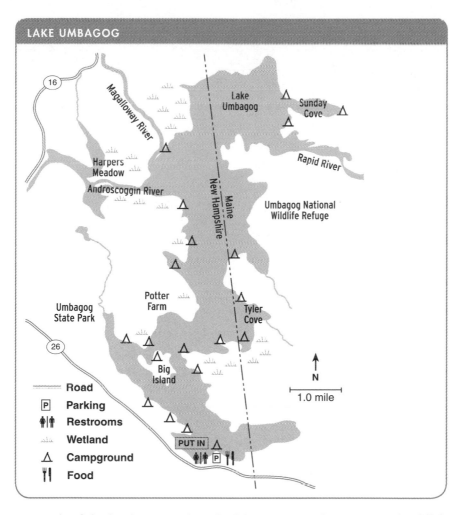

16

Magalloway River

Lake
Umbagog

Sunday
Cove

Rapid River

Harpers
Meadow

Androscoggin River

New Hampshire

Maine

Umbagog National
Wildlife Refuge

Potter
Farm

Umbagog
State Park

Tyler
Cove

26

N

1.0 mile

Big
Island

Road

P Parking

Restrooms

Wetland

Campground

Food

PUT IN

Much of the land surrounding the lake is managed as a national wildlife
refuge. Aside from the state park and campground land on the southwest
shore and a handful of hunting camps and cottages on the southern end, the
lake is wild country that feels larger than its 12 square miles. You will feel as
if you could explore this place forever. To truly experience the beauty of Lake
Umbagog, plan an overnight canoe or kayak camping trip. There is truly nothing like sitting by a crackling fire on the shoreline, listening only to the calls of
the loons echoing across the water. (Note: Dogs are allowed at the base campground area but are prohibited on beaches and many of the remote campsites;
contact park for additional information.)

Long lakes can become treacherous in high winds and waves on the lake
can swamp a kayak or canoe. Start your paddling early in the morning when
the water is glassy smooth and plan to be off the water before the afternoon

winds pick up. Mosquitoes and blackflies can be overwhelming here in mid-summer, so bring bug spray. Our favorite time to visit is in spring or fall when the bugs are not as plentiful.

The easiest place to start your adventure is from the campground, where you'll find boat docks, ample parking, water, and food at the campground store. Remote campsites must be reserved in advance at 877-647-2757 or nhstateparks.org. Here are some of our favorite places on Lake Umbagog.

Big Island
Home to many fine secluded campsites, Big Island is a perfect destination for young families who want to get into the backcountry but don't want to paddle all day to get there. Just a couple miles from the put-in at the campground, this island is permanently protected by the Society for the Protection of New Hampshire Forests.

Tyler Cove
Teeming with wildlife, Tyler Cove has many fine west-facing campsites for beautiful sunsets. A couple of nice sandy beaches make excellent day-trip destinations, with picnic spots galore. Campsites 21–23 are especially nice for families with small children as they have nice sandy beaches.

Androscoggin River and Magalloway River
The Magalloway River flows into the lake and the Androscoggin River flows out of the lake at virtually the same place. The maze of wetlands, floating bogs, river channels, and ponds here is a paddler's paradise, and you can spend hours exploring this prime migratory bird habitat. Be sure to bring a highly detailed USGS map as the many channels and coves can be very confusing.

Sunday Cove and Rapid River
At perhaps the most remote corner of the lake, camping on Sunday Cove and paddling up the remote Rapid River are both very wild experiences.

PLAN B: Milan Hill State Park on NH 16 offers yurt accommodations and some short hikes. You can also trek up Magalloway Mountain (Trip 41) in Pittsburg to enjoy the fire tower with panoramic views of the North Country.

NEARBY: Errol has a diner and a couple convenience stores, and Berlin and Gorham to the south offer many fine options including pizza, delis, Chinese food, and ice cream stands.

Trip 41

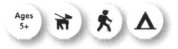

Magalloway Mountain

This hike in a remote corner of the state offers mountaintop views from a fire tower, waterfalls, swimming holes, and the chance to spend the night in a fire warden's cabin!

Address: Magalloway Mountain Road, Pittsburg
Difficulty: Moderate
Distance: 2.0 miles, round-trip.
Hours: No posted hours
Fee: Free for day use; contact Lake Francis State Park for cabin rental fees
Contact: New Hampshire Division of Forests and Lands, 603-271-2214, nhdfl.org/new-hampshire-state-lands/state-owned-reservations; Lake Francis State Park (cabin rental; nearby camping), 603-538-6965, 877-647-2757 (reservations), nhstateparks.org/explore/state-parks/lake-francis-state-park.aspx
Bathrooms: Pit toilet at the parking lot
Water/Snacks: None
Maps: USGS Magalloway Mountain quad
Directions by Car: From the intersection of NH 45 and US 3 in downtown Pittsburg, drive north on US 3 for 11.6 miles past First Connecticut Lake. Take a right on Magalloway Road and immediately set your car's trip meter to zero; these are active logging roads and are not signed. Logging trucks have the right of way on this road, so go slow and give them plenty of room. Continue on this road, crossing over the Connecticut River, staying straight at 1.1 miles, bear left at 2.9 miles, and at 5.3 miles take a right on Magalloway Mountain Road. Continue straight at the intersection at 6.3 miles. At 8.3 miles the road will end at a turnaround and the trailhead (45° 4.125′ N, 71° 10.310′ W). It is highly recommended that you have a *New Hampshire Atlas and Gazetteer* (DeLorme) with you to help navigate the maze of logging roads in this area.

This remote hike is truly off the beaten path, and you will have hundreds of miles of North Country wilderness to yourself—along with the moose, coyotes, foxes, bears, bobcats, and beavers that call this place home. A world away from the beaches of the seacoast, the heavily traveled trails of the White Mountains, and the calm waters of the Lakes Region, this special corner of the state offers a true wilderness experience. Given the distances to get here, it is best experienced as a multiday trip, staying in campgrounds nearby at Lake

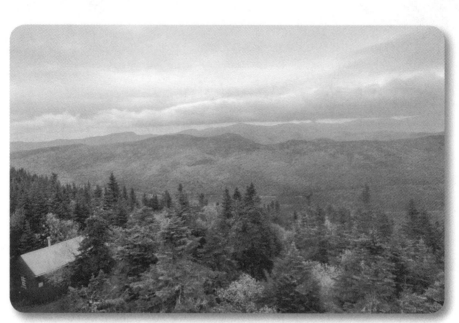

The North Country woods seem to stretch forever from the top of the Magalloway fire tower. (Photo courtesy Patricia Ellis Herr)

Francis, Coleman, or Deer Mountain state parks—or in the cabin on the summit of Mount Magalloway itself!

Mount Magalloway is the only prominent peak in the Connecticut Lakes Region with a trail leading to the top. At the summit, a decommissioned fire tower offers panoramic views of these dense forests and streams, and you can now stay in the former backcountry fire warden's cabin for a taste of what it must be like to live deep in these wild woods.

Starting at the parking area, simply continue up the short but steep Coot Trail that served as the access road for the fire wardens who lived at the fire tower at the summit (see Trip 45, Fire Towers).

After 1.0 mile of hiking through the dense North Country forest of balsam fir, birch, and spruce trees, you reach the summit and the five-story-high fire tower with commanding views of the entire region. To the south, the Presidentials rise on the horizon. To the northwest, Lake Francis and First Connecticut Lake are clearly visible, creating the headwaters of the mighty Connecticut River that flows south between New Hampshire, Vermont, Massachusetts, and Connecticut, before emptying into Long Island Sound, 410 miles away. Behind the warden's cabin there is a short, signed trail that leads to open ledges on the east side of the summit for views into Maine.

If you'd like to stay in the cabin, contact Lake Francis State Park ahead of time. You'll have to pack in supplies, but the cabin sleeps four and has a woodstove, a kitchen, an outhouse, and a small living area.

PLAN B: Nearby Garfield Falls (45° 1.794′ N, 71° 7.019′ W) is one of the most majestic falls in the state, and if you've come this far north, it is worth the extra effort to find it. The 40-foot falls are in a deep granite gorge buried deep in the North Country forests, and the swimming hole at the base is excellent. It is highly recommended that you have a *New Hampshire Atlas and Gazetteer* (DeLorme) with you to help navigate the maze of logging roads in this area.

From the Magalloway Mountain parking area, head back 3.0 miles to Magalloway Road. Reset your trip meter to zero here, and turn right on Magalloway Road (away from US 3). After 3.2 miles, stay straight, and bear right at 4.0 miles. At 5.4 miles, stay straight. At 6.8 miles, you reach a large gravel pull-off surrounded by boulders and a small outhouse; this is the parking area for Garfield Falls. Park and walk a few yards on the road to the trail on the left. A very short hike leads you to the falls and swimming holes. Explore upstream and downstream of the main fall for a beautiful gorge and smaller pools.

NEARBY: Pittsburg offers basic sundries and has a good steak house and pizza pub as well.

Section 4

Southern
New Hampshire

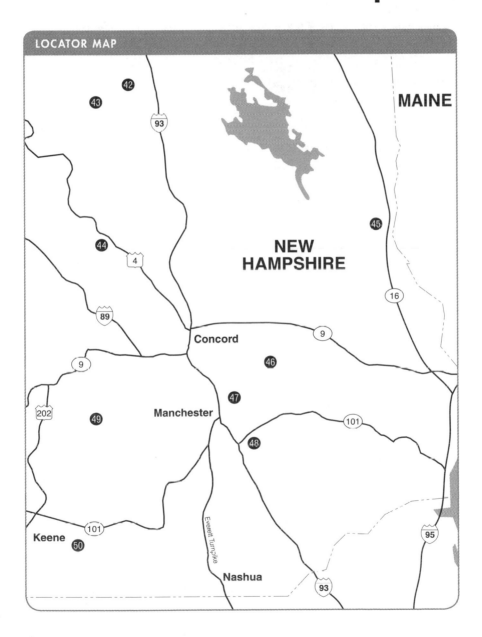

LOCATOR MAP

MAINE

NEW
HAMPSHIRE

42

43

93

44

4

89

45

16

9

Concord

46

9

47

202

49

Manchester

101

48

101

95

Keene

50

Everett Turnpike

Nashua

93

Trip 42

Mount Cardigan

Enjoy a quintessential hike through a mossy ravine and a long, gradual climb to spectacular views, with side trips to a beautiful waterfall and swimming holes.

Address: Shem Valley Road, Alexandria
Difficulty: Challenging
Distance 5.6 miles, round-trip
Hours: No posted hours
Fee: Free for day use; contact Appalachian Mountain Club (AMC) for lodge and campsite fees
Contact: Cardigan State Park, nhstateparks.org/explore/state-parks/cardigan-state-park.aspx; AMC Cardigan Lodge and Campsites, 603-466-2727 (reservations), outdoors.org/cardigan
Bathrooms: At AMC Cardigan Lodge
Water/Snacks: At AMC Cardigan Lodge
Maps: USGS Mount Cardigan quad; *Southern New Hampshire Trail Map*, Map 2: D5–D3 (AMC)
Directions by Car: From the intersection of NH 3A and NH 104 in Bristol, take Route 3A north for 2.1 miles. Turn left onto West Shore Road at the blinking light (a stone church is on the far left corner). Go 1.9 miles, then continue straight onto Cardigan Mountain Road as West Shore Road turns right. In 1.0 mile, turn left onto North Road. In 1.0 mile, turn right onto Washburn Road. In 200 yards, bear right onto Mount Cardigan Road. Follow Mount Cardigan Road for 3.6 miles, and stay left at the intersection with Brook Road. Take Shem Valley Road 1.5 miles to Cardigan Lodge (43° 38.966′ N, 71° 52.660′ W).

Though it requires one of the most challenging hikes in this book, Mount Cardigan is a great destination for those ready for a true mountain expedition. The trip has so much to offer families: a gentle grade, waterfalls, swimming holes, caves, a jaw-dropping summit with views into Vermont and Maine, and amenities at AMC's cozy Cardigan Lodge and Campsites. Home-cooked meals are available to guests at the lodge or the campground, including fresh-baked breads daily, homemade soups, and hearty entrees, all served family-style in a rustic dining hall. (Note: Dogs are allowed on-trail, but not at the lodge or campsites.)

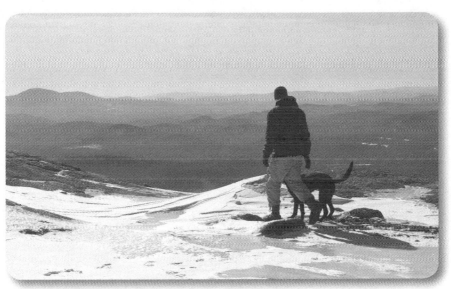

Wide-open skies and granite slabs greet you on the summit of Cardigan.
(Photo courtesy of New Hampshire Department of Parks and Recreation)

From Cardigan Lodge, take Holt Trail to its intersection with Manning Trail, and veer left to stay on Holt Trail. Veer left at Grand Junction (1.1 miles) onto Cathedral Forest Trail (also known as Holt Clark Cutoff Trail). Follow this 0.6 mile to Clark Trail and turn right.

Clark Trail climbs steadily through a northern hardwood forest of sugar maples and birches. It emerges from the trees onto a rocky ridge with excellent views. From June through August, the delicious low-bush blueberries in this area are ripe for the picking. Mount Cardigan's distinctive open granite summit is in the subalpine zone, where the conditions are so harsh that plants can't grow much higher than waist height and the scrawny trees that do survive are called "krummholz," which is German for "crooked wood." Notice the forests of miniature spruce trees that have been stunted by the extreme weather conditions on this exposed ridge.

The expanses of open granite slabs on the summit (2.6 miles) are awe-inspiring, and you will want to leave plenty of time to explore, eat lunch, and soak in the views of the Green Mountains, Mount Kearsarge, Mount Monadnock, and Ragged Mountain to the south and the White Mountains to the north.

From the summit, continue on the loop by following Mowglis Trail for 0.5 mile to the summit of Firescrew, the northern shoulder of Mount Cardigan. In between these two peaks, a 0.25-mile spur path leads to some interesting rock overhangs and small caves known as the Grotto. From the summit of Firescrew, take Manning Trail for 2.5 miles down to the Cardigan Lodge.

PLAN B: If you're staying at Cardigan Lodge or Campsites, visit beautiful Welton Falls. From Cardigan Lodge, take Lower Manning Trail 1.1 miles to the 15-foot falls and their excellent swimming holes. On the way, you can stop at the Fowler River's countless swimming holes, so make a day of it by bringing a picnic and working your way down the river to the falls and back. There are some nice pools farther downstream from the falls as well, so continue exploring if you have the time.

Nearby Wellington State Park on Newfound Lake offers the largest freshwater beach in New Hampshire. The 59-mile Northern Rail Trail stretches from Franklin to Lebanon through the Mascoma River Valley, passing farms, covered bridges, lakes, and bogs. Bring your bikes to Cardigan for this outstanding side trip on a section of this trail!

NEARBY: Nearby Canaan on NH 4 offers pizza, delis, and some basic restaurants. The Cardigan Mountain Orchard at 1540 Mount Cardigan Road offers fresh-picked apples and baked goods.

Trip 43

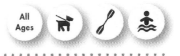

Grafton Pond

This paddler's paradise boasts islands, miles of wildlife habitat to explore, and a virtually undeveloped, protected shoreline.

Address: Grafton Pond Road, Grafton
Difficulty: Easy
Distance: 1.0–3.0 miles
Hours: No posted hours
Fee: Free
Contact: Society for the Protection of New Hampshire Forests, 603-224-9945, forestsociety.org/ourproperties/guide/?block=48
Bathrooms: Portable toilet in summer months
Water/Snacks: None
Maps: USGS Enfield Center quad; forestsociety.org/ourproperties/guide/048/048_map.pdf
Directions by Car: From NH 4A in Enfield Center, follow NH 4A south for 2.2 miles. Take a left onto Bluejay Road/Grafton Pond Road. Continue for 0.9 mile, and then bear right at the fork onto Grafton Pond Road. Continue another 0.9 mile and make a right. The state-maintained boat access will be on your left 0.25 mile (43° 34.794′ N, 72° 2.727′ W).

This is one of our favorite family adventure destinations in New Hampshire. A trip to this small but secluded pond is a treat, and the kids will love the countless islands to explore, blueberry picking, and marshy areas with wildlife.

Although only 300 acres, the pond feels much bigger thanks to its dozens of small islands, long and narrow inlets, and lack of motor- and speedboats. Motors are limited to 6 HP on this lake, which keeps motor traffic and wakes to a minimum. The water is clear and swimmable. Many islands have nice rocky granite slabs that heat up in the sun and make for great "beaches" in which toddlers can wade and splash. Some are shadier and better for those hot days when you want to keep out of the sun. The smallmouth bass fishing is excellent, too, making it a great place to introduce youngsters to the joys of freshwater fishing.

Visiting Grafton Pond is always special, but arrive at or soon after sunrise to see the pond at its best. The mist hovers over the glassy smooth water,

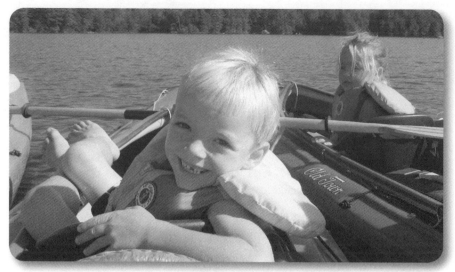

*While you're out on Grafton Pond, find an island or shoreline
to explore, take a dip, and maybe catch a fish or two.*

and quiet blankets the surrounding forest as you paddle into the heart of this wild pond.

Wildlife is most active at dawn and dusk, and your chances of seeing a beaver, fox, or moose are highest at the twilight hours. The loons are most active at night. Come early or stay late to experience their magical calls, but be sure to leave them plenty of room so as to not disturb this threatened species. Along the north shore of the lake, beaver dams dot the marshy shoreline, and you may see one of these industrious creatures stockpiling woody material to make repairs to their lodge or store food on the lake bottom (see Trip 10, About Beavers). We have also seen otters here, which is a real delight.

PLAN B: The Montshire Museum of Science in nearby Norwich, Vermont, is an excellent rainy day option. With hands-on activities, wildlife exhibits, and a freshwater aquarium, this place is definitely worth checking out.

The 59-mile Northern Rail Trail stretches from Franklin to Lebanon through the Mascoma River Valley, passing farms, covered bridges, lakes, and bogs. Bring your bikes for an outstanding side trip while visiting Grafton Pond. You can also plan to stay at AMC's Cardigan Lodge in Alexandria; visit outdoors.org/lodging for more information.

NEARBY: Enfield and Canaan both offer basic eateries. Lebanon, a little farther to the west on NH 4, offers a wide array of dining options including pubs, ice cream stands, and farm stands. Canoe and kayak rentals are available at outfitters in New London and Wilmot Flat.

Trip 44

Ages 5+ $ 🐕   🥾   🏊

Mount Kearsarge

A short hike up this craggy little summit offers commanding views of the Connecticut River Valley, Mount Monadnock, Green Mountains, and, on clear days, Boston!

Address: Winslow State Park, 475 Kearsarge Valley Road, Wilmot
Difficulty: Moderate
Distance: 2.75 miles, round-trip
Hours: Gates open 8 A.M.–6 P.M., seasonally
Fee: $4 adults, $2 children ages 6–11
Contact: 603-526-6168, nhstateparks.org/explore/state-parks/winslow-state-park.aspx
Bathrooms: At the trailhead
Water/Snacks: Water available at the trailhead
Maps: USGS Andover quad; *Southern New Hampshire Trail Guide*, Mount Kearsarge (AMC)
Directions by Car: From the intersection of US 3 and US 4 in Boscawen, head west on US 4. After 15.2 miles, stay left when NH 11 splits from US 4. Proceed on NH 11 another 2.4 miles, and turn left on Old Winslow Road. In 1.0 mile, turn left onto Kearsarge Mountain Road. After 0.6 mile, stay right on Kearsarge Mountain Road and continue for another 0.8 mile to the Winslow State Park picnic area (43° 23.393′ N, 71° 52.080′ W).

Small, mighty, wild-feeling Mount Kearsarge's bare, windswept summit offers some of the finest views in southern New Hampshire. This 2.75-mile loop has a steep 1.0-mile ascent that can be challenging but doable for small kids and a gradual 1.75-mile descent. If you have a choice, always ascend steep sections and descend gradual sections, as it is easier on your body and safer as well. The kids will thank you!

Winslow Trail climbs steeply up the northern ridge of the mountain from the picnic area. There is 1,000 feet of elevation gain here in 1.0 mile, so you are going up 1 foot for every 5 feet you walk! There are many finely constructed rock staircases up this steep section of trail. The reward at the top of this 2,890-foot mountain is the spectacular panoramic views from the open craggy summit. The White Mountains are visible to the north, the Green Mountains

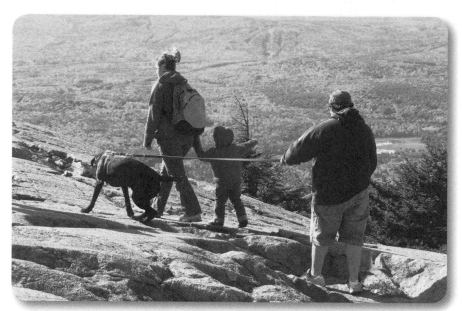

Dogs are welcome on many New England trails, and keeping them on a leash in high-use areas such as Mount Kearsarge protects native wildlife and other visitors. (Photo courtesy of New Hampshire Department of Parks and Recreation)

to the west, Mount Monadnock to the south, and the Merrimack Valley to the east. Mount Kearsarge may not be the highest mountain, but the relatively flat area around it helps reinforce the impression that it's much higher than it is.

After a summit picnic, descend the gradual slopes of Barlow Trail. While it is almost twice as long as the Winslow Trail, the trip on Barlow Trail feels much faster as you are walking down a gentle grade, rather than climbing down a steep set of rock staircases.

PLAN B: If the weather is bad or you want a shorter route up Mount Kearsarge, drive to Rollins State Park on the south side of the mountain and follow its winding road that makes it to within a half-mile of the summit (43° 22.741′ N, 71° 51.514′ W).

The excellent Pollards Mills swimming hole is worth the drive (about 40 minutes north, 43° 20.333′ N, 72° 10.412′ W). Well-tended gardens, picnic tables, and a short nature trail surround this little Shangri-La of waterfalls and swimming holes. Located on private property, the owner encourages respectful visitors to come enjoy this natural wonder.

NEARBY: Nearby New London is a small town with a wide array of eateries and pubs, including the Flying Goose Brew Pub which offers live music.

These iconic backcountry structures have played a vital role in our nation's history and even our literature. Fire towers were originally constructed on tops of mountains so that rangers and fire wardens could spot and report forest fires. In the twentieth century, many towers were staffed by backcountry fire wardens who actually lived at the top of the fire tower. Equipped with a small kitchen, a bed and a desk, these mountaintop perches attracted an especially wild breed of outdoorsperson who gravitated toward this solitary and remote work. Some famous writers even formulated their masterpieces high up in fire towers: Ed Abbey, Jack Kerouac, and Norman Maclean all spent months living in these secluded hermit holes.

Today, fire wardens keep watch over the forests by airplane more often than by tower. But across the country, thousands of these historic structures still stand, giving hikers excellent views of the landscape. Nothing beats the thrill of getting to a high-mountain peak and climbing five stories to see the land just fall away beneath you in a dizzying 360-degree panorama!

One great way to experience New England's fire towers is to take part in the New Hampshire Division of Forest and Lands's Fire Tower Quest program. Hike to five of the fifteen fire towers in New Hampshire, document it on the division's information sheet, send it in and receive a Fire Tower Quest patch! For more information, visit nhdfl.org/fire-control-and-law-enforcement/fire-towers.aspx.

By far the most exciting way to experience a fire tower is to actually stay at one—which you can do at New Hampshire's Mount Magalloway (see Trip 41). After hiking to the summit of the mountain, you will find the old ranger's cabin next to the tower complete with bunks and a small kitchen.

Hikes in this book that lead to a tower:
- Mount Battie, ME (Trip 12)
- Douglas Mountain, ME (Trip 17)
- Pleasant Mountain, ME (Trip 19)
- Mount Magalloway, NH (Trip 41)
- Mount Cardigan, NH (Trip 42)
- Mount Kearsarge, NH (Trip 44)
- Blue Job Mountain, NH (Trip 45)
- Elmore Mountain, VT (Trip 72)

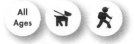

Blue Job Mountain

Hike to see a fire tower and some of the greatest views in the region—and explore an abandoned mica mine!

Address: First Crown Point Road, Farmington
Difficulty: Easy
Distance: 1.0 mile, round-trip
Hours: No posted hours
Fee: Free
Contact: New Hampshire Division of Forests and Lands, nhdfl.org
Bathrooms: None
Water/Snacks: None
Maps: USGS Baxter Lake quad; *AMC White Mountain National Forest Map & Guide*, I12 (AMC)
Directions by Car: From the junction of NH 28 and NH 126 in Barnstead, head east on NH 126 toward Strafford. About 0.5 mile after passing Strafford Town Hall, veer left on NH 202A. In 3.6 miles turn left on First Crown Point Road. Proceed for 4.6 miles past the Blue Job Mountain State Forest sign to the parking area on the right (43° 19.929′ N, 71° 6.908′ W).

This could be the perfect trip for the youngest hikers. A short trail leads to commanding views and a fun trip up a fire tower at the top. Blue Job Mountain can be very busy on weekends, so if you are looking for a more secluded experience, try visiting on a weekday afternoon after school or for an early evening supper on the summit. Always bring a headlamp if you plan to be out in the late afternoon or early evening.

From the trailhead and parking lot, ascend the steeper, right-hand trail; you'll come down the mountain by taking the longer yet easier-to-descend trail on the left. The entire route is marked with orange blazes, both on trees and on the rocky ledges. There are many side trails and older routes, so be sure to keep the blazes in sight.

At 0.4 mile the rocky path approaches a small lookout on the right. This is a good spot to take a water break, but don't stay too long because the summit is just ahead. Continue on to the summit where you will find a working fire tower (0.5 mile). While the views from the summit are good, climb the tower's

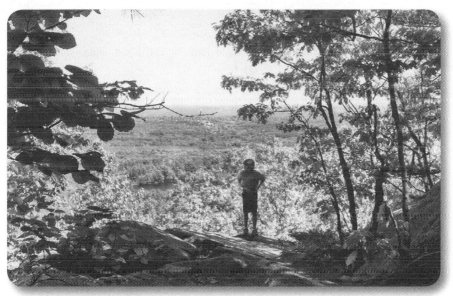

A southern New Hampshire gem, Blue Job Mountain and neighboring Parker Mountain offer rare views in this flatter part of the state.

stairs to look out over a giant swath of New Hampshire. Blue Job Mountain has a high degree of prominence (the vertical rise above surrounding land), so the views are excellent. On a clear day, you can see the Atlantic Ocean to the east and Mount Washington to the north.

After taking a break or a picnic at the summit, continue on the loop following the orange blazes to the southwest. Another small ledge with a communications tower (0.6 mile) has nice views to the west. This is a great alternative break or picnic spot if the summit is crowded when you visit. Continuing on, follow the orange blazes down the hill. At the trail junction at the base of the mountain, head left. The path crosses a couple of bridges and muddy areas, so leave time to explore the brooks and aquatic life along this woodland section of the trail.

PLAN B: If you are in the area and if the kids (and you) have the energy, plan to stop at Parker Mountain and the nearby abandoned mica mine. From Blue Job Mountain, follow First Crown Point Road back to NH 202A and turn right. Continue on to Strafford and turn right on NH 126. Follow NH 126 west through Strafford and the road will begin to rise up to a small notch. The parking area will be on the left just before the height-of-land, approximately 2.5 miles past the junction with NH 202A in Strafford (43° 17.583′ N, 71° 9.617′ W)

Spencer Smith Trail ascends Parker Mountain from this trailhead. Either head up 0.3 mile for some very good ledgy outcrops with great views to the east (including getting a great view back to Blue Job Mountain), or continue onward to the true forested summit (1.1 miles).

To reach the abandoned mica mine from the trailhead, cross NH 126 and walk down the shoulder to the east (downhill) for about 75 feet. A tongue of asphalt heads down into the woods, and a primitive narrow trail descends away from the road. The trail heads downhill, swings left, and then right again. After about 660 feet, the route reaches a steeper section and the first piles of mica tailings. Continue down these piles and to the right to reach the main mine.

Rather than a shaft mine with dangerous tunnels that could collapse, the site is a forested hillside in which miners dug a deep open trench to search for the minerals over 100 years ago. Water trickles down the 50-foot walls and lush plants grow in the shade. You can spend hours sifting through piles of mica or finding new deposits in the rock faces themselves.

NEARBY: Chichester on NH 28 and Center Barnstead on NH 126 both have general stores with basic picnic supplies and ice cream, while Epsom and Concord offer a full array of eating options. The Chichester Country Store is famous for its homemade doughnuts.

WHY DID MINERS DIG FOR MICA?

Mica is fun to find in the woods. Kids and adults alike can spend hours finding the biggest, clearest pieces to treasure. But hundreds of years ago, mica was used for very practical purposes, and miners could make a living digging for this valuable mineral.

Mica was primarily used like glass in the days when Europeans were beginning to settle New Hampshire. In colonial times, glass was very expensive and very difficult to make and transport across long distances, so early settlers used it around the house for anything we use glass for today. It has a very high resistance to heat and is close to fire-proof, so it was used to make peepholes into woodstoves and for lanterns as well. The biggest pieces would be connected together to make windows for a house.

Mica is still used around the world today in electronic devices like smartphones, as well as filler for drywall and roof shingles. That's why roof shingles sparkle when you look at them closely!

Trip 46

Beaver Pond

Take a scenic hike to backcountry ponds, complete with swimming and blueberry picking, in New Hampshire's second largest state park.

Address: Bear Brook State Park, Allenstown
Difficulty: Easy
Distance: 1.5 miles, round-trip hiking
Hours: Park gates open Monday–Friday, 9 A.M.–8 P.M., Saturday–Sunday, 8 A.M.–6 P.M., seasonally
Fee: $4 adults, $2 children ages 6–11; contact park for campground fees
Contact: Bear Brook State Park, 603-485-9874 (day use), 603-485-9869 (campground), nhstateparks.org/explore/state-parks/bear-brook-state-park.aspx
Bathrooms: At campground
Water/Snacks: At campground
Maps: USGS Candia quad; nhstateparks.org/uploads/pdf/Bear-Brook_Trail-Map.pdf
Directions by Car: From the intersection of US 3 and NH 28 in Allenstown, head northeast on NH 28 for 3 miles to the large sign for Bear Brook State Park on the right. Take a right here onto Deerfield Road. In 3.2 miles, take a right on Podunk Road. Cross a brook and veer left at the fork in the road. Continue for 2.8 miles on this park road until you reach the campground. Park near the campground office and head left past the ball field on your right to campsite 26 and the beach on Beaver Pond (43° 6.949′ N, 71° 19.695′ W)

Bear Brook State Park is an oasis of ponds, marshes, and deep pine forests in a corner of the state that is becoming increasingly populated. As New Hampshire's second largest state park (after the largely undeveloped Pisgah State Park), Bear Brook has something for everyone, including peaceful hiking, ponds and marshes, top-notch cross-country skiing, archery courses, fishing ponds, swimming holes, and an increasingly popular mountain bike culture. When you are deep in this serene 10,000-acre preserve, you will never guess

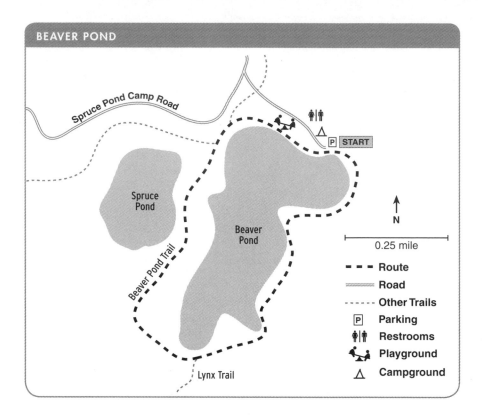

BEAVER POND

Spruce Pond Camp Road

Spruce
Pond

Beaver
Pond

Beaver Pond Trail

Lynx Trail

P START

N

0.25 mile

- - - Route
==== Road
----- Other Trails
P   Parking
🚻   Restrooms
🛝   Playground
⛺   Campground

that the busy urban centers of Manchester and Concord are less than a half hour away!

Like state parks throughout New England and the rest of the country, Bear Brook owes its stone picnic pavilions, hand-dug swimming holes, and campgrounds to President Franklin Roosevelt's Civilian Conservation Corps (CCC) of the 1930s. Bear Brook was even home to two CCC-era camps where hundreds of men were housed and fed as they completed projects throughout New Hampshire. One of those camps is still used today by the modern-day incarnation of the CCC, the New Hampshire Conservation Corps.

Beaver Pond is a great place to start exploring this park, although many other great options exist and are listed in the Plan B section of this trip. From the campground, walk toward campsite 26 at the end of the campground road. Proceed out across the nice sandy beach (stopping for a swim if you like). Continuing on, the road enters a forest of large white pines mixed with a beech and hemlock understory. The forest floor here is soft and fragrant, with a thick mat of pine needles. Hugging the edge of the pond to your right, the road passes some boulder slabs along the pond shore that make an excellent rest stop and swimming spot.

Continuing on around the pond, the road crosses a narrow isthmus of land that separates Beaver Pond from nearby Spruce Pond. This is a very wet area, with a lot of good blueberry picking. The route also passes a finely constructed timber bridge, complete with a bench that's perfect for sitting quietly and scanning for wildlife. Beaver, deer, moose, bobcats, coyotes, and dozens of kinds of birds call this marshy wildlife paradise home. The best time to see wildlife here is in the early morning or as the sun is setting.

Continue along the pond back through the campground to the parking area. The campground rents canoes on Beaver Pond for a small fee, and the playground in the campground makes an excellent stop before you head home.

PLAN B: No matter the season, it's difficult to run out of things to do in Bear Brook State Park. Hike to remote and marshy Smith Pond and its shelter and fire pit via Broken Boulder Trail. When the weather is warm, enjoy a dip in the excellent swimming hole at Catamount Pond on Deerfield Road as you head out of the park. When it's cold, ice skate on Spruce Pond and Beaver Pond. Because of the limited snowmobile traffic, the ice is often smooth and makes for a great winter pond exploration. The park is also an idyllic cross-country ski destination, with mostly ungroomed backcountry trails. The rolling, generally flat terrain makes it a great spot for beginners and families. Skiers and snowmobilers use separate trails. Recommended kid-friendly cross-country ski trails are Broken Boulder, Pitch Pine, and Bobcat.

NEARBY: The traffic circle in nearby Epsom has a few eateries, and nearby Concord has many options, including sushi, pizza, and excellent bagel shops and delis.

Trip 47

Dubes Pond

This serene pond offers rich wildlife viewing, islands, and coves.

Address: NH 27 (between Farwood Lane and Rowes Corner Lane), Hooksett
Difficulty: Easy
Distance: 2.0–4.0 miles, round-trip
Hours: No posted hours
Fee: Free
Contact: New Hampshire Fish and Game, 603-271-3421, wildnh.com
Bathrooms: None
Water/Snacks: None
Maps: USGS Manchester North quad; cyclingnewengland.blogspot.com/2011/05/
   rockingham-recreational-trail-new.html
Directions by Car: From I-93, Exit 9N, and head north on NH 28/US 3 for
   2.1 miles, and then turn right on NH 27/Whitehall Road. Follow NH 27/
   Whitehall Road for 2.6 miles until you see the pond on your left. Launch
   boats on the pond side, then move your car to the large parking lot across the
   road from the pond (43° 3.966′ N, 71° 23.819′ W).

Dubes Pond is one of those special places that begs to be explored. It is a mere
ten minutes from the hustle and bustle of downtown Manchester, yet out in
the far reaches and coves of this secluded pond you feel as if you are in the
North Country of Maine or Quebec. It is a haven for wildlife, and it would be
surprising if you didn't see herons, snapping turtles, painted turtles, big water
snakes, beaver, foxes, or ducks during your visit. This is an absolutely great
place to play wildlife bingo, as you are sure to see so many animals. Visit Dubes
Pond in early season (April and May) or late season (October and November)
to avoid the vegetation and waterlilies that grow so thick you can barely paddle
through them. Before or after summer, though, the exploring is phenomenal.
There is even a "secret" pond that you can find, complete with a heron rookery.

Starting at the put-in, paddle your way out to the dozens of islands that
dot this 111-acre pond. The western shore has a few homes on it, but most are
hidden in the trees. The eastern shore is completely undeveloped and makes
for interesting shoreline paddling amid the white pines and granite boulders

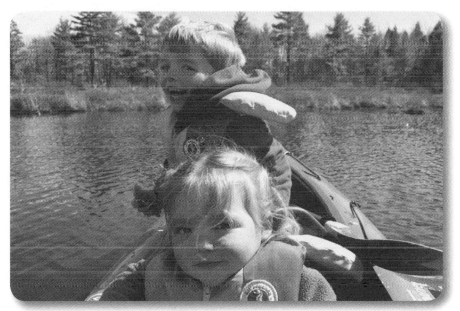

With a double kayak or a full-sized canoe, you can fit the entire family for a paddling adventure. Or split into two or more boats for added independence once the kids are older.

dotting the shoreline. Find an island to explore and have a picnic. Just always be aware and respectful of wildlife, as birds use these islands to lay and hatch their eggs in spring. There are also several beaver dams on the pond, all with secret entrances below the waterline (see Trip 10, About Beavers).

Continuing on away from the road and toward the left, the pond begins to close in. Follow a narrow channel northward for up-close wildlife viewing. If you are ambitious, you can follow this small channel all the way to a small natural dam. A short portage over the dam brings you to the secluded Hinman Pond and a heron rookery. The herons nest in these dead trees; their giant nests high up in the air are a sight to see.

PLAN B: Nearby Bear Brook State Park (Trip 46) offers many hikes, rides, and paddles. An excellent swimming hole at Catamount Pond on Deerfield Road in Allenstown offers clear and cool swimming on a hot day.

NEARBY: Elm Street in downtown Manchester has everything from Vietnamese and Ethiopian food to Irish pubs, so take a walk down here for a surprising eclectic dining scene. The nearby Golden Rod Drive-In on Candia Road has great ice cream. Canoe and kayak rentals are available at outfitters in Raymond, Concord, and Manchester.

Trip 48

Rockingham Recreational Rail Trail

This idyllic bike path leads you past lakes and streams, and through dense forests in Manchester.

Address: NH 28 Bypass/Londonderry Turnpike (between Auburn Circle and Dechenes Road), Auburn
Distance: 2.0–20.0 miles, round-trip
Difficulty: Easy–Moderate
Hours: No posted hours
Fee: Free
Contact: New Hampshire State Parks, 603-271-3254, nhstateparks.org/explore/bureau-of-trails/rockingham-recreational-trail-portsmouth.aspx
Bathrooms: None
Water/Snacks: None
Maps: USGS Manchester North, Candia, and Mount Pawtuckaway quads
Directions by Car: Take I-93, Exit 7 and head east on NH 101. After 1.5 miles, take Exit 1 for NH 28 Bypass. Turn right on NH 28 Bypass/Londonderry Turnpike. At the traffic circle, continue straight to stay on NH 28 Bypass. Take an immediate left into the parking area for Massabesic Lake (43° 0.218′ N, 71° 23.419′ W).

Rockingham Recreational Rail Trail is nestled in one of the more urban corridors of New Hampshire, connecting Manchester to Great Bay on the Seacoast. This segment offers excellent opportunities for biking, swimming, fishing, and wildlife observation. Since the trail runs so close to water, bring bug spray to keep the mosquitoes at bay. The surface of the path as you continue east is variable, so road bikes are not recommended past the first mile from the parking area on this route. Jogging-type strollers with large wheels should be fine, but leave the umbrella strollers at home. The trail is a fun challenge for anyone with mountain, touring, or just sturdy kids' bikes. (See Getting Started when you're considering your ideal turnaround point.)

From the parking area at Massabesic Lake, follow the bike path along the northern shore. While you may want to go for a dip here, this is the primary water supply for Manchester and swimming is not permitted. The trail winds

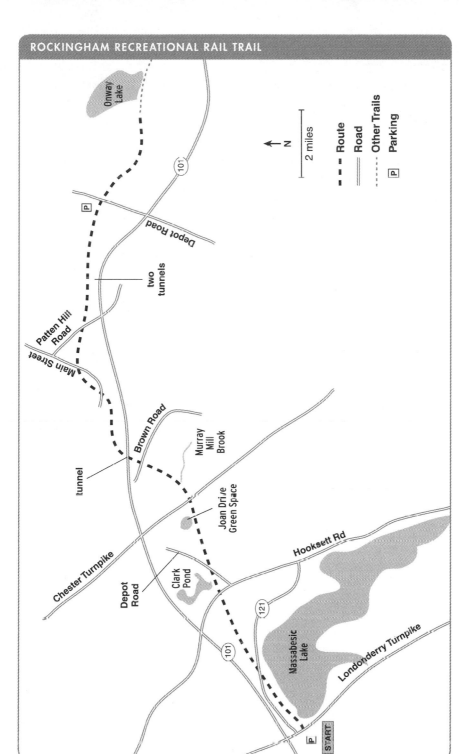

Onway Lake

101

N

2 miles

- - - Route
——— Road
········ Other Trails
P Parking

Depot Road

P

two tunnels

Patten Hill Road

Main Street

Brown Road

Murray Mill Brook

tunnel

Joan Drive Green Space

Chester Turnpike

Hooksett Rd

Depot Road

Clark Pond

121

Massabesic Lake

Londonderry Turnpike

101

P START

peacefully along the northern shore for a mile or so, always with the lake in view.

The path continues east past the lake through forests and residential areas but crosses no major roads thanks to several tunnels. You do, however, cross dozens of tributary streams and skirt along the edge of multiple wetlands. Take your time and try sitting quietly along the shore to get the best view of the abundant wildlife. Loons populate these undeveloped shorelines, and ospreys visit in spring. Even bald eagles are known to winter near Massabesic Lake. The trail crosses a couple of ponds on causeways built for the railroad that once frequented this route and connected Portland, Manchester, Boston, and New York.

Onway Lake (10 miles from Lake Massabesic) is a turnaround point if you have the stamina for a 20-mile round-trip. There are good picnic and swimming spots here, and even a rope swing!

PLAN B: The nearby New Hampshire Audubon Massabesic Center in Auburn hosts nature programs, wildlife viewing, and a 5-mile network of trails on its lakeside property.

NEARBY: Elm Street in downtown Manchester has everything from Vietnamese and Ethiopian food to Irish pubs, so take a walk down here for a surprising eclectic dining scene. The nearby Golden Rod Drive-In on Candia Road has great ice cream.

Trip 49

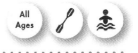

Nubanusit Lake and Spoonwood Pond

Explore this crystal clear lake to see a bald eagle nest, ride a thrilling rope swing, and take a small portage to a hidden pond with backcountry campsites.

Address: Kings Highway, Nelson
Difficulty: Easy
Distance: 2.0–4.0 miles, round-trip
Hours: No posted hours
Fee: Free
Contact: Harris Center for Conservation Education, 603-525-3394, harriscenter.org; New Hampshire Fish and Game, wildnh.com
Bathrooms: None
Water/Snacks: None
Maps: USGS Peterborough North quad
Directions by Car: From the intersection of NH 123 and NH 137 in Hancock, continue west on NH 123 for 2.1 miles. Turn left onto Hunts Pond Road and continue for 0.5 mile onto Kings Highway. Pass Hunts Pond on your left and continue for another 1.1 miles to the boat access road that turns off on the left (42° 59.834′ N, 72° 2.688′ W).

Nubanusit Lake's geology and topography make for the clearest waters we've seen on any lake in New Hampshire. While it can get busy on a hot summer day, it is a big lake and there are secluded corners to which you can retreat. And, if you are willing to do a 100-foot portage, you can paddle Spoonwood Pond, which offers all of the beauty, clear water, and granite slabs of Nubanusit Lake without any motorboats.

From the boat ramp, paddle along the right-hand (northern) shore. Much of the land along here is undeveloped and protected as conservation land managed by the local land trust, the Harris Center for Conservation Education. The lake's clear waters allow you to see straight through to the sandy bottom, with hardly a trace of vegetation typically found in New Hampshire's lakes and ponds. This is caused by the depth of the water (96 feet in Nubanusit Lake and 70 feet in Spoonwood Pond) as well as a lack of wetlands

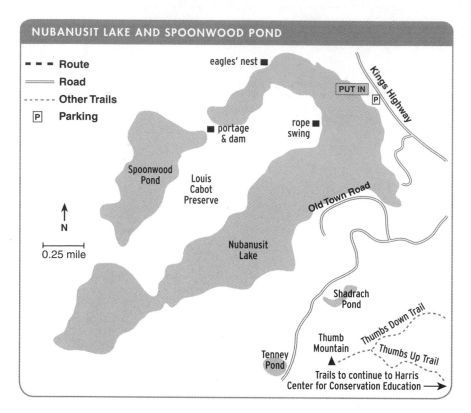

and marshes surrounding the lake, creating a habitat with very low biological productivity and clear and clean water. Bring your snorkels and masks for hours of freshwater exploration in these sparkling clear waters. Look for the circular sand nests that sunfish create on the sandy bottom. The lake offers excellent trout fishing as well.

Continue along the shore and look for the bald eagles' nest, high up in some pines. Be sure to steer clear and give them plenty of room as human disturbance will inhibit their success here. Eagles stopped nesting in the state in 1949 and didn't return until 1989. Nubanusit Lake was one of the first places that they returned to and they are still nesting and breeding successfully here.

On the far northwest corner of Nubanusit Lake, look for a small earthen dam and the short portage into Spoonwood Pond (1.2 miles from the put-in). This small pond has no road access and is only reachable by the adventurous souls who paddle and portage there. The quiet, protected waters are perfect for families, and you may see turtles, otters, and foxes. A couple of reservation-only backcountry campsites are nestled on its shores. Only sponsors of the Harris Center for Conservation Education may make reservations. If you plan ahead and wish to contribute to this land trust, this can be a unique backcountry camping experience right in southern New Hampshire.

From Spoonwood Pond, follow the right-hand shore to a thrilling rope swing directly across the lake from the boat ramp (1.0 mile).

PLAN B: The Harris Center for Conservation Education is just down Kings Highway from the boat ramp. The center's property offers trails to Thumb Mountain and views of several nearby ponds. The Harris Center also has educational programs, camps, and green building tours.

NEARBY: Nearby Peterborough is a charming New England village full of restaurants featuring a range of cuisine, including delis, pizza pubs, Italian, and fine dining. It also has some excellent ice cream stands. The nearest canoe and kayak outfitters at the time of publication were in Concord and Manchester.

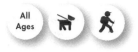

Gap Mountain

A short hike leads to blueberry picking and an open summit that offers views to Mount Monadnock and the Green Mountains of Vermont.

Address: Bullard Road (between NH 124 and Old Mill Road), Jaffrey
Difficulty: Easy
Distance: 2.6 miles, round-trip
Hours: No posted hours
Fee: Free
Contact: Society for the Protection of New Hampshire Forests, 603-224-9945, forestsociety.org/ourproperties/guide/?block=18
Bathrooms: Portable toilet at trailhead
Water/Snacks: None
Maps: USGS Troy quad; forestsociety.org/ourproperties/guide/018/018_map.pdf
Directions by Car: From the intersection of US 202 and NH 124, head west on NH 124 for 6.0 miles to Bullard Road. Turn left on Bullard Road and proceed for 0.5 mile to a driveway to the trailhead parking on the left (42° 49.773′ N, 72° 7.826′ W).

Situated just south of the legendary Mount Monadnock, Gap Mountain rises from the valley floor and offers a more tranquil and less strenuous experience for families with kids than its big brother to the north. An easy 1.3-mile hike leads to open summit views that allow you to see directly across the valley to the granite slab slopes of Mount Monadnock. A busy summer day here may see a few dozen hikers cross over the summit, but nearby Mount Monadnock sees 500 to 1,000 hikers on the same day, with 125,000 hikers summiting every year. What Gap Mountain lacks in size, it makes up for in solitude, ease, and natural beauty.

Owned entirely by the Society for the Protection of New Hampshire Forests (SPNHF), the Gap Mountain Reservation has been preserved by various landowners since the early 1900s. These landowners saw the incredible beauty of this spot and realized its development potential, but opted instead to donate their land to SPNHF for perpetual conservation, wildlife habitat, and recreation for the public. As you hike through the soft understory of this forest,

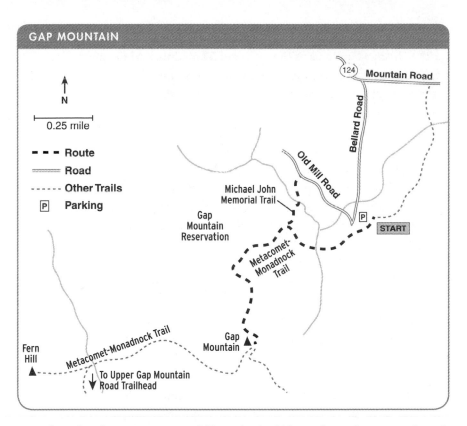

N

0.25 mile

- - - **Route**
===== **Road**
------ **Other Trails**
P **Parking**

124 **Mountain Road**

Bellard Road

Old Mill Road

Michael John
Memorial Trail

Gap
Mountain
Reservation

Metacomet-
Monadnock
Trail

P

START

Fern
Hill

Metacomet-Monadnock Trail

Gap
Mountain

To Upper Gap Mountain
Road Trailhead

consider what this property would have looked like without the essential work of local land trusts and conservation groups.

From the parking lot, stop at the kiosk for valuable information. Head out on the trail to the right of the kiosk to immediately reach Metacomet–Monadnock Trail, where you will turn right. This trail will be marked with white blazes on trees and rocks the entire way up—make sure you are always following the white blazes, as there are several unmarked trails in the area that can be confusing.

The trail crosses several stone walls, a legacy of the former uses of this property. It was not uncommon in the 1800s for entire mountains to be deforested and made into pasture. These rocks mark the edges of old fields, from which farmers and their horses pulled the stones to create the walls. As you hike across the walls, you are hiking across pieces of history.

After crossing over a lovely babbling brook, the trail starts its ascent to the summit. The footpath is laid out well and the ascent is gradual for the entire hike. About halfway up, several small caves on your left are worth exploring!

Near the summit, the forest starts to thin, and the trail enters an excellent blueberry habitat. Your pace will surely slow here as you pick your way up the trail (at least, when the blueberries are ripe). A clearing ahead is the North

Summit, one of three on Gap Mountain, but the one with the best views. Look for the Green Mountains to the west and Monadnock to the north. "Monadnock" is an Abenaki word for "mountain that stands alone." Standing on this summit, it's clear why that monolithic mountain earned its name. Hike down the way you came.

PLAN B: Be sure to check out the amazing stone arch bridge over the Ashuelot River on the way to Keene. Head west on NH 124 for 6.4 miles, then 2.8 miles west on NH 101; the bridge is on your left. At 50 feet over the river surface, it is one of the highest stone arch bridges ever built in the state. Today it is part of the Cheshire Rail Trail, and its unmortared rock joints make it popular with rock climbers.

Head to nearby Nubanusit Lake and Spoonwood Pond (Trip 49) for excellent paddling, swimming, and camping. Nearby Gilson Pond Campground in Monadnock State Park offers car camping and remote camping options. Peaceful Greenfield State Park in Greenfield is home to excellent camping, an undeveloped lake, a sandy swimming beach, nature trails, and canoe and kayak rentals.

NEARBY: Both Peterborough to the east and Keene to the west have a wide variety of surprisingly cosmopolitan dining options, along with numerous ice cream stands.

Section 5

Southern Vermont

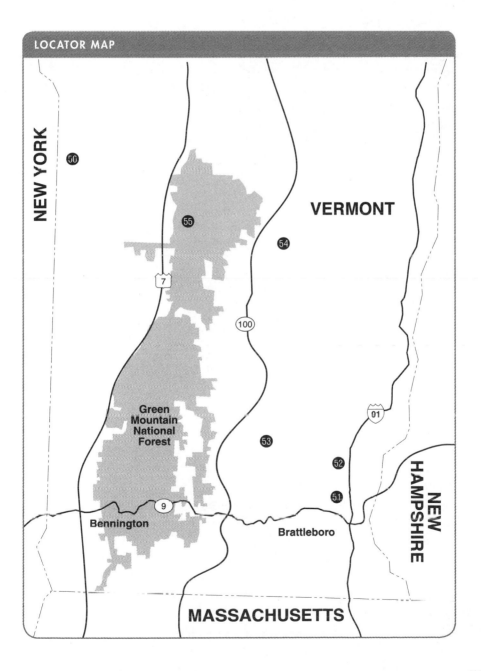

LOCATOR MAP

NEW YORK

50

VERMONT

55

54

7

100

Green
Mountain
National
Forest

01

53

52

51

9

Bennington

Brattleboro

NEW
HAMPSHIRE

MASSACHUSETTS

Trip 51

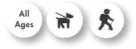

Putney Mountain

A gently graded trail through hardwood forests to a grassy mountaintop with expansive views of southern Vermont make this a perfect hike for even the smallest legs.

Address: Putney Mountain Road (between Banning Road and Grassy Brook Road), Putney
Difficulty: Easy
Distance: 1.2 miles, round-trip
Hours: No posted hours
Fee: Free
Contact: Putney Mountain Association, putneymountain.org; Windmill Hill Pinnacle Association, 802-869-2071, windmillhillpinnacle.org
Bathrooms: None
Water/Snacks: None
Maps: USGS Putney and Westminster West quads; windmillhillpinnacle.org/images/maps/maps_pdfs/PMA_Trails.pdf
Directions by Car: From the intersection of VT 5 and Westminster Road in Putney, drive west on Westminster Road. After 1.1 miles, turn left on West Hill Road. Proceed for 2.3 miles and turn right on Putney Mountain Road. Continue 2.2 miles to the hairpin curve and the trailhead parking area on the right (42° 59.806′ N, 72° 36.024′ W).

Putney Mountain could be the perfect first hike for the youngest hikers. With a 1.2-mile loop, easy grades, interesting trees to climb, and a fantastic view from the grassy summit, it simply adds up to a fantastic experience for small children. It is quite short and easy, so older kids might find it a bit unchallenging, but a great outing and picnic spot regardless. If you combine it with a stop at a local swimming hole, a lunch outing, or a visit to Putney's apple orchards (see Plan B), you've got a fabulous day for everyone.

Putney Mountain Town Forest is part of a string of preserved ridge-top conservation lands that stretch northward to the Pinnacle (Trip 52) and beyond. Overall, there are 20 miles of ridgeline that have been permanently preserved for recreation and wildlife. Starting in August and lasting into December, thousands of birds of prey migrate through this corridor, some to places

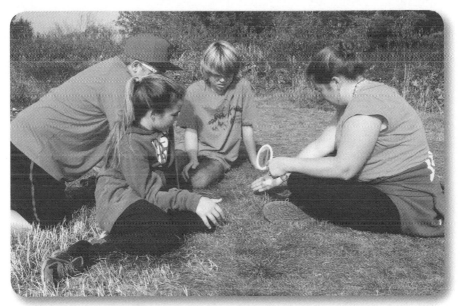

Take time to explore even the smallest parts of nature on this easy and short hike to Putney Mountain's grassy summit.

as far away as South America, and Putney Mountain is renowned for its view of this spectacular sight.

From the parking lot, stay to the left and take West Cliff Trail (0.1 mile, yellow blazes). Winding gently through peaceful hemlock groves, the trail meets a stone wall, which is a reminder that this land was once cleared and used as pasture lands. Imagine the views from these hills 150 years ago without a single tree on them! The beautiful grassy summit is just beyond the stone wall (0.6 mile). Look for New Hampshire's Mount Monadnock to the east and the Green Mountains to the west. See if you can pick out the ski trails on Stratton Mountain or spot a hawk flying overhead.

At the summit, follow blue blazes to Ridge Line Trail (white blazes) that will loop you back to the trailhead (1.2 miles). Along the way back, you will come across the famous Elephant Tree. Everyone will have fun climbing the unusual trunk that runs parallel to the ground for a good 15 feet or so. If you look at it and squint your eyes, you can imagine that this horizontal trunk just might resemble an elephant's trunk.

PLAN B: Green Mountain Orchards in Putney is a great place to pick up fresh apples, pick your own blueberries, eat some cider doughnuts, or go for a hayride.

Swimming at Pikes Falls in nearby Jamaica will be a highlight of your trip. With a 10-foot rock slide, waterfall, large swimming hole, and rocky beach, you could spend the entire day here. From Putney Mountain, head west on Putney Mountain Road for 2.3 miles, and turn left onto Brookline/Grassy Brook Road. Follow this for 1.0 mile, cross the West River, and turn right onto Upper River Road. Follow this for just under a mile where it merges onto VT 30. Follow VT 30 for 12.5 miles into Jamaica and turn left on South Hill Road. After 200 feet, fork right onto Pikes Falls Road. Follow this for 2.3 miles where Pikes Falls Road continues right and cross a bridge. Keep going to the wide pull-off on the left after another 2.4 miles. Park and head down to the river to the left. It is highly recommended that those looking for swimming holes use these rough directions in combination with the *Vermont Atlas and Gazetteer* (DeLorme).

NEARBY: Putney has a great selection of restaurants and delis, including the historic and newly rebuilt Putney General Store, which serves excellent sandwiches and picnic fare. Stop by Curtis' BBQ on US 5 to enjoy live music, a playground, and, of course, piles of barbecue served out of a blue school bus in a tranquil park-like setting.

Trip 52

The Pinnacle

Follow a gently winding, moderately graded trail through maple groves to a sunny, west-facing summit with expansive views and a stone overnight shelter.

Address: 1026 Windmill Hill Road North, Westminster
Difficulty: Easy
Distance: 3.0 miles, round-trip
Hours: No posted hours
Fee: Free
Contact: Windmill Hill Pinnacle Association, 802-869-2071, 802-463-9226 (shelter reservations), windmillhillpinnacle.org
Bathrooms: None
Water/Snacks: None
Maps: USGS Westminster West quad; windmillhillpinnacle.org/pages/trailmaps/area_maps/areamap_south.html
Directions by Car: From the intersection of VT 5 and Kimball Hill Road/Westminster Road in Putney, follow Kimball Hill Road/Westminster Road, which becomes Westminster West Road, west for 6.9 miles to the village of Westminster West. Turn sharply left onto West Road at the church. Follow West Road just over 0.9 mile and turn right on Windmill Hill Road North. The Holden Trailhead is 1.0 mile ahead on this road on the right (43° 3.379′ N, 72° 34.006′ W).

Moderate and gently graded, this hike is filled with natural history wonders, stone walls, and ancient foundations to explore. The route passes through some beautiful open maple groves and emerges on the 1,683-foot summit with wide-open views to the west and a stone overnight shelter. The land is owned by the Windmill Hill Pinnacle Association, which has protected more than 1,800 acres of land stretched out over this 20-mile ridge in southeastern Vermont and is one of many small community-based land trusts in New England preserving land for wildlife, conservation, and recreation.

From the Holden Trailhead, head west past the artistically inspired iron gate. Proceed up Holden Trail for 0.5 mile past some fine examples of colonial farmhouse foundations, abandoned wells, and stone walls. You will also spot many large wolf trees along the way. Turn right at the first trail intersection

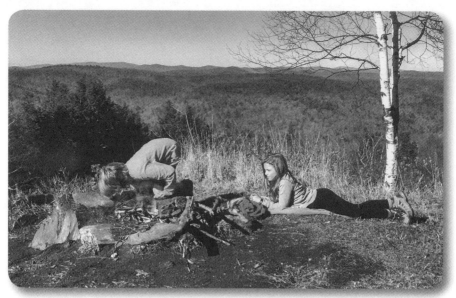
The fire ring located at the Pinnacle shelter provides a
great place to hone those fire-starting skills!

and continue up Holden Trail. The trail begins to climb a bit here, but never too steeply. Near the summit, the path cuts through a fine mature maple grove with an open, grassy understory. This rare grove likely evolved this way as the result of a single wolf tree. Only sedges and grasses grow below the maples now, and the wide-open forest understory is a rare and beautiful sight.

After 0.9 mile, turn left on Pinnacle Trail; your destination is just ahead through the trees. The trail emerges onto the Pinnacle, a gorgeous open summit with a stone and timber overnight shelter. Kids will have a blast exploring the shelter and climbing up to the large sleeping loft. The shelter is free to stay in and open to the public, but reservations through the Windmill Hill Pinnacle Association are required. Soak in the views and the sunshine—you can see five different ski areas and many of Vermont's highest peaks from here. See if you can spot them all.

Return the way you came for a 3.0-mile round-trip.

PLAN B: Green Mountain Orchards at 130 West Hill Road in Putney is a great place to pick up fresh apples, pick your own blueberries, eat some cider doughnuts, or go for a hayride. Also nearby are the rock slides and pools of Pikes Falls in nearby Jamaica (see Trip 51).

NEARBY: Putney has a great selection of restaurants and delis, and even a not-to-be missed barbecue joint. The historic and newly rebuilt Putney General

Store, first built in 1769, offers excellent sandwiches and picnic fare. Stop by Curtis' BBQ on US 5 to enjoy live music, a playground, and, of course, piles of barbecue served out of a blue school bus in a tranquil park-like setting.

WOLF TREES

By observing the woods around us, we can figure out clues about the history of the places we visit. In the 1800s, as much as 80 percent of the land in New England had been turned into pasture and meadow, leaving only 20 percent forested. Farmers made a good living raising sheep for meat and wool, but in the 1900s other materials came into fashion and much of the pasture land was abandoned, allowing the forest to return to New England.

Today when you walk through the woods you can see some clues that the land once was used as sheep pasture—one of which is a wolf tree. These trees once grew in the middle of pastures, drinking in as much sunshine as they wanted, allowing them to spread out and grow big and bushy. Now that years and years have passed, the forest has often grown back around the wolf trees. The new trees, however, are tall and skinny in comparison and help observant hikers easily see the old wolf trees. See how many wolf trees you can find along this trail.

Trip 53

West River Trail and Hamilton Falls

After biking along the scenic West River, a peaceful woodland hike leads you to the base of 125-foot Hamilton Falls, and a swimming hole in the West River awaits your return.

Address: Jamaica State Park, 48 Salmon Hole Lane, Jamaica
Difficulty: Easy
Distance: 4.0 miles, round-trip, biking; 2.2 miles, round-trip, hiking
Hours: 10 A.M.–sunset, May 9 through Columbus Day weekend
Fee: $3 adults, $2 children ages 4–14
Contact: Jamaica State Park, 802-874-4600, vtstateparks.com/htm/jamaica.htm; Friends of the West River Trail, westrivertrail.org
Bathrooms: At Jamaica State Park Campground
Water/Snacks: At Jamaica State Park Campground
Maps: USGS Jamaica quad; vtstateparks.com/pdfs/jamaica_trails.pdf
Directions by Car: From the intersection of VT 100 and VT 30 in East Jamaica, continue west on VT 100/VT 30 for 3.1 miles to Depot Street in Jamaica. Turn right on Depot Street and follow it for 0.4 mile, continuing on a bridge over the West River into Jamaica State Park. Make an immediate left after the bridge onto Salmon Hole Lane and continue to the end of this short road and the large parking area (43° 6.343′ N, 72° 46.403′ W).

This trip combines three great activities into one awesome day: biking along West River Trail to Hamilton Falls Trail, then hiking to Hamilton Falls, then swimming in the refreshing Salmon Hole on your way back. Mountain and hybrid bikes will serve you best on the gravel trail.

From the parking area, continue on to West River Trail which is managed by the Friends of the West River Trail. Their mission is to complete and maintain this 36-mile trail, which follows the route of a historic rail line that ran here at the turn of the nineteenth century. Many sections are complete; others are still in development. (Check the Friends' website for full details.) The section described here is complete and nicely graded as it follows the contour

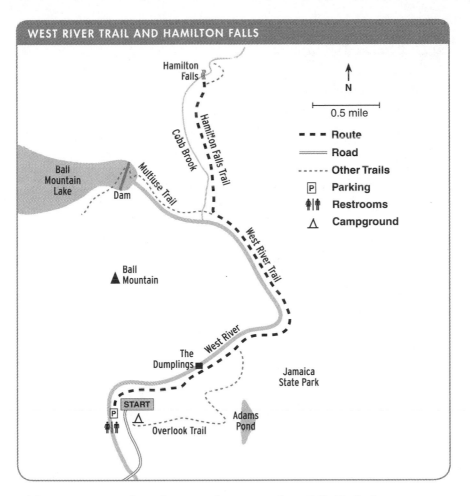

Hamilton
Falls

N

0.5 mile

- - - Route
=== Road
----- Other Trails
P Parking
Restrooms
Campground

Cobb Brook

Hamilton Falls Trail

Multiuse Trail

Ball
Mountain
Lake

Dam

West River Trail

Ball
Mountain

The
Dumplings

West River

Jamaica
State Park

START

P

Overlook Trail

Adams
Pond

of the West River. Along the 2.0 miles to Hamilton Falls Trail, there are many spots to stop and play in the river or cast a line for fish.

Hamilton Falls Trail joins on your right, just before the bridge over Cobb Brook. Lock your bikes to a tree and head off up Hamilton Falls Trail on foot. Your young ones will feel as if they are on an epic adventure while using multiple means of transportation to reach their destination. At 1.1 miles, the short and steep trail reaches a spur trail to the falls; turn left here.

Hamilton Falls is one of the most spectacular of Vermont's hundreds of waterfalls. Over the course of its 125-foot plummet, it has created numerous potholes, gorges, and a great wading pool at the base with plenty of sunshine and a great picnic spot. We highly discourage families with young children from venturing above the lower pool; the rocks and pools above are very steep, slippery, and can be quite dangerous.

Returning the way you came, grab your bikes and head back to the campground. Take a dip in the Salmon Hole, which is just off of the parking area where you started. Look for the stairs leading down to the river, and a lazy pool with a sandy beach and sunny lounging on a hot summer day.

PLAN B: The campground at Jamaica State Park has a nice playground so stop by for a few minutes of outdoor fun. Many trips in this book are nearby (Trips 51, 52, 54, and 55), making this park an excellent place to use as base camp for your southern Vermont explorations.

With a 10-foot rock slide, waterfall, large swimming hole, and rocky beach, you could spend the entire day at Pikes Falls in Jamaica. See details and directions in Trip 51.

NEARBY: Brattleboro is surprisingly cosmopolitan and has a wide variety of eating establishments, pubs, and delis, and Jamaica has a small assortment of restaurants and stores, and a coffee house.

Trip 54

Lowell Lake

Peaceful, flat water; beaver dams; sunning turtles; and islands perfect for exploration and picnics make this a great first family paddle.

Address: 260 Ice House Road, Londonderry
Difficulty: Easy
Distance: 1.0–3.0 miles
Hours: 10 A.M.–sunset
Fee: Free
Contact: 802-824-4035, vtstateparks.com/htm/lowell.htm
Bathrooms: None
Water/Snacks: None
Maps: USGS Londonderry quad; vtstateparks.com/pdfs/lowell.pdf
Directions by Car: From VT 11 in Londonderry, turn onto Lowell Lake Road. In 0.5 mile, turn right at T intersection. Park entrance is just up the hill (43° 13.360′ N, 72° 46.344′ W).

The shallow, 102-acre lake will feel manageable and safe for young kids, and the waves never build up except in the most extreme conditions. Explore four of the lake's five islands and its completely undeveloped shoreline.

The southernmost island is private property, but the rest are open to the public. The state park has transported picnic tables to some of the islands, making for civilized lunch spots. The average depth of the lake is 20 feet, meaning that the water warms up quickly in spring and makes for warm swimming. It is also home to warm-water pond fish such as bass, perch, and pickerel, so bring along your rods! Everyone will be intrigued by the prolific beavers at this lake. There are a couple of large beaver dams on the lake that perfectly showcase the ingenuity of "nature's engineers" (read more about beavers in Trip 10).

A 3.5-mile trail also loops around the lake. It is marked by blue blazes and is mostly flat and very easy, if not a bit wet in spots.

PLAN B: Londonderry is an outdoors paradise with many hiking, swimming and paddling options. Try the nearby Bromley Mountain (Trip 55) or head a little south for a hike at the Pinnacle (Trip 52). The multiple pools of Butter-

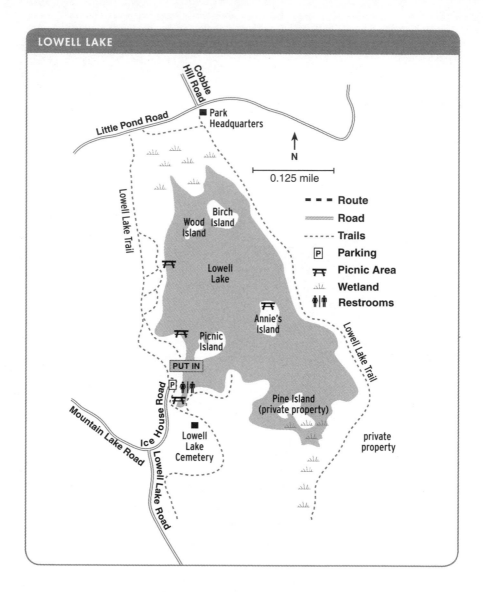

Route
Road
Trails
P **Parking**
Picnic Area
Wetland
Restrooms

0.125 mile

N

Cobble Hill Road

Little Pond Road

Park Headquarters

Lowell Lake Trail

Birch Island

Wood Island

Lowell Lake

Annie's Island

Lowell Lake Trail

Picnic Island

PUT IN

Ice House Road

Mountain Lake Road

Lowell Lake Road

Lowell Lake Cemetery

Pine Island (private property)

private property

milk Falls on Buttermilk Falls Road in Ludlow (43° 26.118′ N, 72° 43.609′ W) make for a great post-hike swim. With multiple pools to choose from, and some good jumping spots, everyone will enjoy an adventure here.

NEARBY: Londonderry has exceptional eating options, including many delis, pizzerias, and higher-end fare as well. Pick up picnic lunch supplies at the farmer's market. The historic Stone Hearth Inn and Tavern on VT 11 in Chester boasts a cozy fireplace, games of pool or darts, pub dinners, and well-known chocolate chip cookie sundaes. Canoe and kayak rentals are available at outfitters in Rawsonville and Bondville.

The state parks in Maine, Vermont, and New Hampshire offer excellent programs to encourage young and old alike to explore their parks. Taking part in all three programs is free, and incentivizes outdoor activities that you may not have tried in the past.

New Hampshire State Parks and The Great Park Pursuit: The Great Park Pursuit is a series of organized events in which family teams participate at various state parks throughout the state. It's a great way to get to know the parks, especially if you're new to outdoor activities and like trying new things in a group setting. Typically events include environmental education and natural history lessons, along with a scavenger hunt in a specific park. For more information, visit nhstateparks.org/whats-happening/great-park-pursuit.

Vermont State Parks and Venture Vermont: It's remarkably easy to take part in this self-guided scavenger hunt for the whole family. Simply download a score sheet from the Vermont State Parks website that lists different outdoors-related challenges for you to complete. Each challenge has a corresponding number of points. To earn them, just document your family completing the activity (usually just by snapping a picture) and return your score sheet to state park headquarters. If you fulfill the goal of reaching 250 points, you receive a special gold coin that gives you free access to all Vermont State Parks for the rest of the year and all of the next!

The real fun of Venture Vermont lies in the wide variety of challenges. Some examples include:

- Sleep under the stars without a tent (10 points)
- Make your own fishing pole with things you find outside (10 points)
- Swim in a lake (5 points)
- Go camping on a bicycle tour (25 points)
- Attend a nature program (15 points)
- Download your score sheet and find more information at vtstateparks.com/htm/venturevt.htm

Maine State Parks and Take it Outside!: The Division of Parks and Public Lands offers the "Take It Outside" program, which offers interpretive events in Maine State Parks. Events are stand-alone, and not part of a series or a contest. Events include nature walks, ice fishing, osprey watch, clamming, and much more. Head to take-it-outside.com for more information about this program.

Trip 55

Bromley Mountain

A moderately graded trail leads you along a brook, past an overnight shelter, and finally to open vistas.

Address: VT 11/30 (between VT 30 and Bromley Forest Road), Winhall
Difficulty: Moderate
Distance: 5.5 miles, round-trip
Hours: No posted hours
Fee: Free for day use; contact Bromley Mountain Ski Resort for chairlift fees
Contact: Green Mountain National Forest, 802-747-6700, www.fs.usda.gov/greenmountain; Bromley Mountain Ski Resort, 802-824-5522, bromley.com, summer.bromley.com
Bathrooms: None
Water/Snacks: None
Maps: USGS Peru quad
Directions by Car: From the intersection of VT 11 and VT 100 in Londonderry, head west on VT 11 for 9.4 miles to the trailhead parking area on the right (43° 14.295′ N, 72° 55.544′ W).

Bromley Mountain makes for an excellent hike for young hikers ready for a walk of 5.5 miles. Unlike older mountain footpaths that take the shortest (and often most challenging) route between two points, this recreational trail follows a more gradual grade that holds up better against erosion than steep slopes. Following the route of the Long Trail, the trip leads to panoramic views on top of the mountain. From Memorial Day to Labor Day, the ski area runs many summer adventure activities and chairlift rides; in May or September through November, the area is less crowded. You can also opt to turn this into an overnight by staying at the new Bromley Mountain Shelter (2.3 miles).

From the eastern end of the parking lot, head east on the Long Trail for about 50 feet, before crossing Bromley Brook. Walk along the brook for 0.9 mile before starting the climb up the mountain. Depending on the season of your visit the hardwood forest will offer many delights on your way up, from beautiful fall foliage to great views when the leaves are long gone.

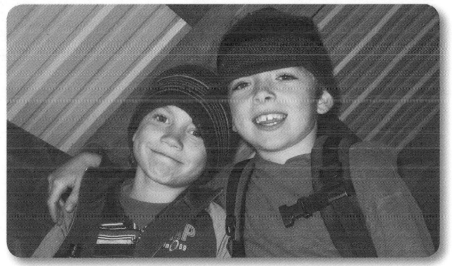
Turn your day hike into a memorable overnight with a stay at Bromley Mountain's shelter.

At 2.3 miles, take the spur trail to visit the shelter. With a loft sleeping area and a picnic table, this is a cozy spot to spend the night. As the shelter is on the well-traveled Long Trail that runs the length of the state from Massachusetts to Canada, other hikers may use the shelter as well. Even if you don't stay, the kids will love to explore and "play house," and it always makes a good spot for a snack break or lunch break.

Further up, the trail emerges from the woods onto the wide and grassy Run Around Ski Trail at the ski area. You are close to the top here! Just turn left and keep climbing to reach a viewing platform with a 360-degree view of the surrounding peaks and valleys. You can see some of Vermont's highest peaks here: Stratton Mountain lies just to the south and Equinox is to the west. Continue down the way you came.

PLAN B: Buttermilk Falls on Buttermilk Falls Road in Ludlow (43° 26.118′ N, 72° 43.609′ W) make for a great post-hike swim. With multiple pools to choose from, and some good jumping spots, everyone will enjoy an adventure here. Lowell Lake on VT 11 in Londonderry is also a great swimming spot.

NEARBY: Both Londonderry and Manchester have exceptional eating options, with many delis, pizzerias, and higher-end fare as well. Excellent farmers' markets in both towns can be a great way to stock up on picnic-lunch supplies. The historic Stone Hearth Inn and Tavern on VT 11 in Chester boasts a cozy fireplace, games of pool or darts, pub dinners, and well-known chocolate chip cookie sundaes.

Trip 56

Ages 5+

Mount Antone and the Merck Forest and Farmland Center

Follow paths and forest roads that meander through farmland and meadows, leading to small mountains with excellent views and backcountry cabins to spend the night.

Address: 3270 VT 315 (Rupert Mountain Road), Rupert
Difficulty: Moderate
Distance: 5.0 miles, round-trip
Hours: Dawn to dusk
Fee: Free for day use; contact Merck Forest and Farmland Center for camping and cabin fees
Contact: Merck Forest and Farmland Center, 802-394-7836, merckforest.org
Bathrooms: At the visitor center
Water/Snacks: At the visitor center
Maps: USGS Pawlet and West Rupert quads; merckforest.org/cms/TrailMap.pdf
Directions by Car: From the intersection of US 7 and VT 30 in Manchester, follow VT 30 west for 1.5 miles and turn right onto Main Street. Make an immediate left onto Bonnet Street to remain on VT 30. Continue on VT 30 for another 8.1 miles and make a left onto VT 315 W/Rupert Mountain Road. Follow VT 315 approximately 2.6 miles to the top of the hill. The driveway to Merck Forest and Farmland Center will be on the left. Proceed 0.5 mile to the parking area and visitor center (43° 16.353′ N, 73° 8.767′ W).

Mount Antone is but one excellent destination at Merck Forest and Farmland Center (MFFC). MFFC also serves as a true, working farm and forest. During your visit to this "land of many uses" you may see any number of activities: timber harvesting, maple sugaring, wildlife habitat restoration and preservation, fruit and vegetable production, livestock production—and of course, recreation. Whether you're exploring MFFC's sustainable farm operation or backpacking through the heart of this 3,100-acre site, you will be delighted to learn about the history of this special place, see amazing vistas, and behold a prime example of successful land that is managed for multiple uses.

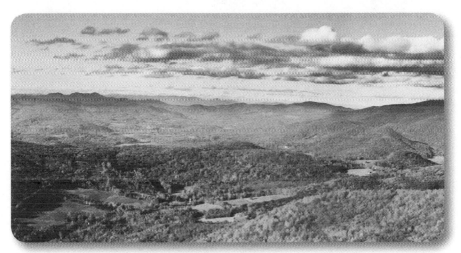

The pastoral mountain landscapes in Merck Forest and Farmland Center are truly breathtaking. (Photo courtesy of Dan Sullivan)

From the visitor center, follow the main arterial trail at MFFC, Old Town Road, for approximately 0.75 mile to the intersection with Antone Road. Along the way, pass the Sap House and a small spur trail up to Page Pond. The route progresses through mixed forests of birch, red oak, and sugar maples. See if you can find evidence of MFFC's sugaring operation here.

Take a right on Antone Road and follow it steadily uphill for another 1.75 miles to the summit of Antone Mountain at 2,600 feet, 900 feet above the visitor center. The views from the summit are great in all seasons, but for the most wide-open views, continue down the shoulder of Mount Antone to the large grassy meadow. Look back to the north to see the farm lying below you, and the pastoral landscape of Vermont and New York. The patchwork of farms and forests is distinctive to this region.

For your return trip, take an interesting side route on McCormick Trail. McCormick Trail leaves Antone Road on the left (4.4 miles). Follow its contours along the edge of an interesting ravine, staying to the right at every intersection to return to Old Town Road. Take a left on Old Town Road and continue for about 0.5 mile back to the visitor center.

PLAN B: There's plenty more to do at MFFC. Pick berries, pet farm animals, swim in a pond, or stay in a cabin or shelter. MFFC even allows dispersed backcountry camping in all seasons, so this makes a great destination for winter camping or backpacking. Besides this excellent hike, there are dozens of great trails and destinations to choose from at MFFC. In winter, you may take a sleigh ride or embark on a moonlit cross-country ski through farm fields on

Burke Trail. Or, you could put together a family-friendly, multiday trek to a series of cabins, shelters, or campsites.

The excellent cabins and shelters at MFFC are a true draw, and are often booked months in advance—especially in winter. Families and groups cross-country ski or snowshoe in to the cabins, towing sleds full of supplies. At the cabins, woodstoves keep the groups warm as they enjoy the tranquility of a snowy night in the Vermont woods. Check availability and make reservations online at merckforest.org.

NEARBY: Nearby Manchester has an excellent collection of restaurants, delis, and pubs to suit any taste.

Section 6

Central Vermont

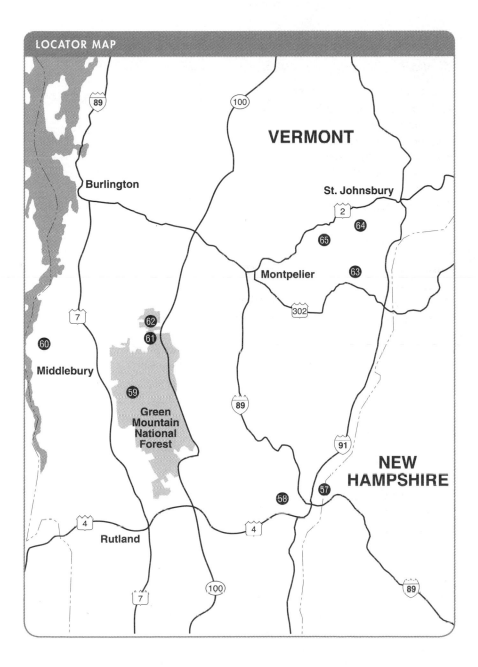

LOCATOR MAP

VERMONT

Burlington

St. Johnsbury

Montpelier

Middlebury

Green
Mountain
National
Forest

NEW
HAMPSHIRE

Rutland

Trip 57

All Ages 🐕 🛶 🏊 ⛺

Connecticut River and Gilman Island

A short and easy paddle on the Connecticut River leads to an idyllic island complete with camping, a rope swing, and great wildlife viewing.

Address: East Wilder Road, Lebanon, NH
Difficulty: Easy
Distance: 2.0 miles, round-trip
Hours: Sunrise to sunset
Fee: Free to paddle and camp; contact Ledyard Canoe Club for cabin and canoe rental fees
Contact: Lebanon Recreation and Parks (boat launch), 603-448-5121, recreation.lebnh.net; Connecticut River Paddlers' Trail, connecticutriverpaddlerstrail.org/node/312; Ledyard Canoe Club (canoe rentals and Titcomb Cabin), (603) 643-6709, dartmouth.edu/~lcc/main/home
Bathrooms: Portable toilet on Gilman Island
Water/Snacks: None
Maps: USGS Hanover quad; *Connecticut River Paddlers' Trail Waterproof Recreation Map and Guide* (Wilderness Map Company)
Directions by Car: *To launch in Hartford, VT*: From I-91 north, Exit 12, take Bugbee Street toward VT 5. After 0.3 mile, turn left onto Hartford Avenue/Taft Avenue/VT 5 and head north for 0.7 mile. Turn right onto Depot Street, then an immediate left onto Norwich Avenue. Take an immediate right onto Passumpsic Avenue. After a couple hundred feet, veer left and then immediately right into the Wilder Dam Boat Launch area, also known as Kilowatt South Boat Landing and Ball Fields (43° 40.485′ N, 72° 18.152′ W). *To launch in Lebanon, NH*: From the intersection of US 4/NH 10 and Main Street/NH 10 in West Lebanon, NH, go north on NH 10 2.1 miles. Turn left onto East Wilder Road. Continue for 0.6 mile, to the obvious gravel pull-off with an information kiosk on the left. A narrow dirt track leads down to a grassy area on the river that makes an ideal cartop boat put-in (43° 40.726′ N, 72° 18.030′ W).

The mighty Connecticut River flows 410 miles from its headwaters near the Canadian border, along the border of New Hampshire and Vermont, through Massachusetts and Connecticut, and eventually into Long Island Sound. In the

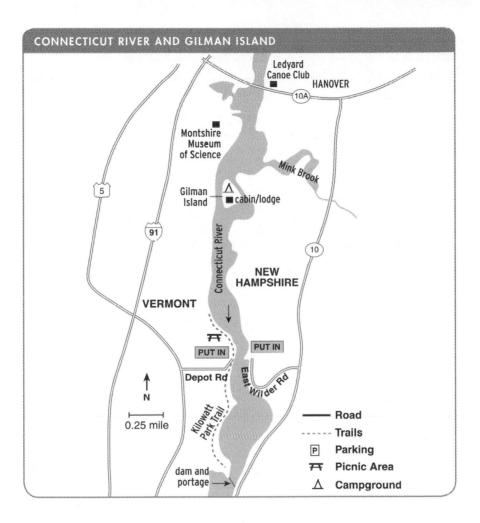

Upper Valley, the river is serene, flat, and dotted with campsites, making this section perfect for families.

This trip is a favorite because of the ease of the paddling, the great campsite on Gilman Island, and close proximity to Norwich's Montshire Museum of Science and the fun college town of Hanover, New Hampshire (see Plan B). The river creates the boundary between New Hampshire and Vermont and access is available from both shores; our preferred access point for this paddle is from the New Hampshire side of the river.

From either put-in, head north up the river. The water is flat here, with no discernible current, as the Wilder Dam just downstream creates a long and narrow lake. On your way to Gilman Island, hug the forested eastern shoreline. You may spot turtles in the sun or even a bald eagle flying overhead. The riverbanks east and west are both protected, so you will never guess that you are less than a mile from bustling towns and an interstate.

The 7-acre Gilman Island is within 1.0 mile of the boat launch and is a perfect spot to stop for a picnic or a swim. Owned and managed by TransCanada, the energy company that manages many of the dams along the Connecticut River, Gilman Island is open for recreational use and now boasts a campsite at the southern end of the island. With ample tentsites, fire rings, and a world-class rope swing, this place is a little piece of paradise. Pack along your tents, sleeping bags, and provisions and plan to stay for a night or two. The camping is first-come, first-served, but there is plenty of overflow space if a group is already there. There is also a small island directly across from Gilman that has space for one family to camp. Gilman Island is also home to the cozy Titcomb Cabin, built by the Dartmouth Outing Club and available for rent to the public; contact the Ledyard Canoe Club for reservations.

From Gilman Island, return the way you came or paddle north as far as you'd like to continue exploring this peaceful section of river.

PLAN B: Paddle another 0.5 mile north from Gilman Island, underneath the Ledyard Bridge to the Ledyard Canoe Club on the east shore. From there, you can land your boat and walk several blocks east to downtown Hanover, New Hampshire, which features pubs, restaurants, farmers markets, shops, and more.

The Montshire Museum of Science in Norwich, Vermont, boasts hands-on activities, wildlife exhibits, a freshwater aquarium, and many special events and programs. Though it's easy to reach by car, you can paddle to the museum from Gilman Island. Just head north for 0.25 mile and look for the small inlet on the left just before the Ledyard Bridge. Land your boat on the shore of the inlet and follow Meadow Walk up to the museum.

NEARBY: Both Hanover and Lebanon, New Hampshire, offer a wide array of dining options including pubs, ice cream stands, and farm stands.

CONNECTICUT RIVER PADDLERS' TRAIL

Thanks to the efforts of many partners, including the Appalachian Mountain Club, the Connecticut River has been at the heart of several initiatives meant to improve access to this essential natural resource. Since the early 1990s, campsites, portage trails, and access points have all been added to make this river friendly to paddlers of all abilities and interests, creating the Connecticut River Paddlers' Trail and earning it the honor of becoming the nation's only National Blueway. For more information on access to and amenities on the Connecticut River, visit connecticutriverpaddlerstrail.org.

Trip 58

Mount Tom

Starting and ending in a town park in quaint Woodstock, Vermont, this pleasant walk features pastoral views, stone bridges, and close proximity to ice cream.

Address: Faulkner Park, Mountain Avenue (between River Avenue and US 4), Woodstock
Difficulty: Easy
Distance: 3.0 miles, round-trip
Hours: No posted hours
Fee: Free
Contact: Woodstock Chamber of Commerce, 802-457-3555, woodstockvt.com/hiking.php; Woodstock Trails Partnership, walkwoodstock.com
Bathrooms: None
Water/Snacks: None
Maps: USGS Woodstock North quad; www.nps.gov/mabi/planyourvisit/upload/Faulkner-Trail.pdf
Directions by Car: From I-89, Exit 1, follow US 4 west for 10.1 miles into downtown Woodstock. Make a slight right onto Mountain Avenue and cross the Ottauquechee River on a covered bridge. In 0.3 mile, just after Mountain Avenue makes a hard left, Faulkner Park will be on your right. Park in the gravel pullouts (43° 37.427′ N, 72° 31.506′ W).

Rather than starting your adventure up this mountain at a remote trailhead, the trek up Mount Tom begins in a quaint New England village, complete with a town green and a bustling commercial scene. After grabbing a sandwich at one of the local delis, take a leisurely stroll up gradual switchbacks to views of the town and river below. This walk combines a gradual grade, excellent views, and proximity to ice cream to make it a great trip for first-timers, including toddlers.

This forest and the town's green spaces have been preserved and restored over the centuries by concerned landowners, various land trusts, and the Billings Park Commission. The extensive trail network and opens spaces within the village of Woodstock are a testament to the power of collaboration and planning for the future. While Mount Tom was completely denuded in the 1800s, it is now home to a mature forest. Many New Englanders are used to

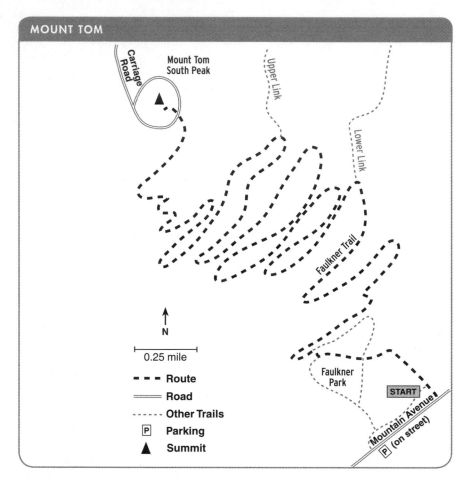

Mount Tom
South Peak

Carriage
Road

Upper Link

Lower Link

Faulkner Trail

N

0.25 mile

- - - Route
===== Road
------ Other Trails
P Parking
▲ Summit

Faulkner
Park

START

Mountain Avenue
P (on street)

young, dense forests filled with understory scrub, but a mature forest left in its natural state—like this one—will most likely have fewer, taller trees that block the sunlight and limit new growth, creating an open, park-like understory that makes for easy travel and great views.

Faulkner Trail departs from the back of Faulkner Park, and the paved path quickly turns to gravel and dirt. This trail traverses *across* the contours of the mountain, climbing gently to the top, rather than just beelining straight up the grade to the summit. This makes for an easy and pleasant stroll for even the fussiest of young hikers. Play a game of Roving Hide and Seek, or try a game of Trail Bingo on your way up (see Trip 21, Games on the Move). The many park benches and a beautiful stone arch bridge give you plenty of interesting places to hide and items to look for. As you ascend, Lower Link Trail and Upper Link Trail will divert to your right—stay left at both of these intersections to reach the summit of Mount Tom. These link trails tie together an extensive network of footpaths that crosses Mounts Tom and Peg, Marsh-Billings-Rockefeller

National Historical Park, the Vermont Land Trust's King Farm, and other green space in Woodstock. Maintained by the Woodstock Trails Partnership, this network of more than 30 miles of trail offers opportunities to hike, cross-country ski, and more. Find more information on Woodstock's trails at nps. gov/mabi/planyourvisit/hiking-trails-walk-woodstock.htm; paper maps are available at the Billings Farm and Museum (see Plan B).

After several more wide switchbacks, the trail reaches a lookout point on your right (1.4 miles). A steep and rocky section a few hundred yards long brings you to the true summit (1.5 miles), wide-open and grassy, with views of Woodstock and the Ottauquechee River Valley. Return the way you came.

PLAN B: The Billings Farm and Museum is both a working dairy farm and an exciting educational experience for the whole family, complete with jersey milk cows, draft horses, chickens, sheep, a farm museum, hands-on exhibits, butter churning, and ice cream. Visit billingsfarm.org for more information.

The Marsh-Billings-Rockefeller National Historical Park also operates out of the visitor center at Billings Farm, with many historical exhibits on conservation in America, along with miles of hiking and cross-country ski trails. Visit nps.gov/mabi for more information.

Twenty Foot, a fun series of swimming holes, is about 20 minutes away. From the intersection of US 4 and VT 106 in Woodstock, follow VT 106 south for 13.7 miles to Tyson Road in Felchville. Take a right and proceed 1.0 mile to the crest of a small hill with a turnoff on the left. Several steep trails lead down to the swimming holes in the North Branch Black River.

NEARBY: Woodstock is full of delis, pizza places, and fine dining to suit any taste.

Trip 59

All Ages

Silver Lake and Falls of Lana

Hike past exceptional waterfalls and swimming holes to a peaceful lake surrounded by backcountry campsites.

Address: VT 53/Lake Dunmore Road (between Kelsey Lane and Indian Trail), Brandon
Difficulty: Easy–Moderate
Distance: 3.2–5.7 miles, round-trip
Hours: No posted hours
Fee: Free
Contact: Moosalamoo National Recreation Area, moosalamoo.org
Bathrooms: At Branbury State Park
Water/Snacks: At Branbury State Park
Maps: USGS East Middlebury quad; moosalamoo.org/maps/silver-lake-area
Directions by Car: From Court Square in Middlebury, head south on US 7 for 6.8 miles to the junction with VT 53/Lake Dunmore Road. Turn left and follow VT 53 for 3.9 miles, past the Branbury State Park entrance, to the Silver Lake trailhead parking on your left (43° 54.034′ N, 73° 3.853′ W).

The Falls of Lana have carved a gorge horizontally through the face of a cliff, with mist rising up from its several cascades. Venture into its secluded swimming holes, and complete your trip with a moderate walk up a babbling brook to a beautiful high-mountain lake, dotted with private backcountry campsites. Make this a weekend trip by staying here or at next-door Branbury State Park's campground on Lake Dunmore. Nestled in the Green Mountain National Forest's Moosalamoo National Recreation Area, this trip is like none other we have found in New England.

From the trailhead, head up the short and steep trail to Silver Lake Trail, a wide carriage road that will serve as your route to Silver Lake (0.1 mile). The path originally served as access to a lakeside backcountry grand hotel that burned down in 1942. The ruins have long since deteriorated and you'd never guess that this was once a bustling mountainside retreat.

Take the left onto Silver Lake Trail. After 0.3 mile it reaches a large, black, overhead pipe that acts as water chute for a hydroelectric plant fed by Silver

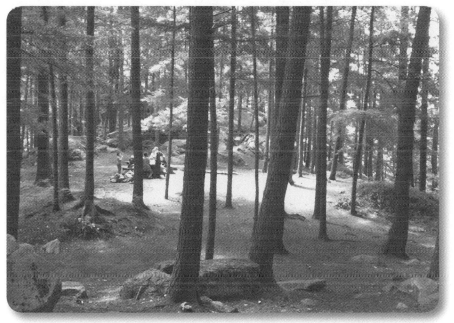

The many excellent campsites along the trail and surrounding Silver Lake make for an easy introduction to backpacking.

Lake. Within 50 feet after crossing under the pipe, a steep, rugged path to the left leads down to the Falls of Lana. Climb down this side trail to a lush grotto with 15-foot rock walls rising up to your left; you can hear the falls ahead here, but you won't be able to see them yet. Turn to your right and walk uphill next to a rock wall. After a hundred yards or so, a break in the rock wall and a narrow access lead to one of the most interesting and secluded swimming holes in Vermont. This swimming hole is perched at the midway point in the Falls of Lana, with spectacular cascades dropping into the pool from above, as well as exiting to a long chute below. The wild and rugged beauty of this secret spot will surely remain in the memories of the young ones for a long time to come. We recommend only swimming here with strong swimmers during periods of low water as current can be strong. Return to the main trail the way you came.

Continuing on Silver Lake Trail, head left and continue uphill along babbling Sucker Brook for 0.5 mile. There are many fine places to swim and wade, so plan to take your time on a hot day. When the trail reaches a bridge and a trail intersection (there are some excellent backcountry campsites here), take a right away from the brook to stay on Silver Lake Trail.

Continue for another 0.8 mile, climbing very gradually on switchbacks. Even though you gain 850 feet of elevation here, you will barely notice it, and we have seen many toddlers running happily up this section of trail. After 0.8 mile, the path reaches the peaceful waters of Silver Lake, surrounded by the foothills of the Green Mountains. Here you have a choice: follow Silver Lake Loop Trail around the lake (an additional 2.5 miles), or simply picnic at the scenic dam. If you choose to skip the loop around the lake, return the way you came (3.2 miles).

If you'd like to stay, Silver Lake's fifteen backcountry campsites are widely spaced along the eastern shore. Adventurous souls may want to tackle this as an overnight trip, as the grades are easy and the 1.6-mile, one-way haul is not too bad. The sites are all widely spaced and private, and many have excellent swimming right from the campsite.

PLAN B: Nearby Branbury State Park on Lake Dunmore offers great camping, a swimming beach, clean facilities, boat rentals, picnic areas, and interpretive programs. From arts and crafts to guided hikes, it is worth a stop to see what's on the schedule. A 1.0-mile hike to Ethan Allen Cave is an interesting side trip. Revolutionary War hero Ethan Allen slept here hiding from English forces. The trailhead leaves from the Branbury State Park campground; ask at the office for directions.

NEARBY: Middlebury is home to some excellent eateries, and closer by, sandwiches and ice cream cones can be found at the Lake Dunmore Kampersville complex.

Trip 60

Snake Mountain

This prominent serpentine monolith rises from Vermont's farmlands, providing excellent wildlife habitat and spectacular hiking.

Address: Mountain Road (between Wilmarth Road and Whitford Road), Addison
Distance: 3.6 miles, round-trip
Difficulty: Moderate
Hours: Sunrise to sunset
Fee: Free
Contact: The Nature Conservancy, 802-229-4425, nature.org/vermont; Vermont Fish and Wildlife Department, 802-828-1000, vtfishandwildlife.com
Bathrooms: None
Water/Snacks: None
Maps: USGS Snake Mountain quad; vtfishandwildlife.com/wma_maps.cfm
Directions by Car: From the intersection of US 7 and VT 22A near Vergennes, head south on VT 22A for 10.4 miles, then turn left on Wilmarth Road. After 0.6 mile, turn left on Mountain Road. In 0.1 mile, turn left into the gravel parking area (44° 2.947′ N, 73° 17.517′ W).

Snake Mountain rises majestically from the rural farmlands of Vermont, towering over the surrounding landscape and providing vital high-country habitat for falcons, deer, coyotes, and even the occasional bear and moose. Mountains that rise above surrounding flatlands like this one are said to have a high degree of "prominence," as there are no other mountains surrounding it to obscure the view. The Nature Conservancy's Williams Woods Natural Area protects about 81 acres of land near the trailhead; as you progress up the trail, you cross into Snake Mountain Wildlife Management Area, overseen by Vermont Fish and Wildlife. No dogs are permitted in Willmarth Woods, so make a plan to leave them at home. The mountain is an island of high county in the surrounding lowlands, which makes habitats it supports very rare and worth protecting.

In the early 1900s, the Grand View Hotel topped Snake Mountain, as was the fashion at the time. Dozens of high-country peaks throughout New England were host to grand, high-class summit hotels that offered overnight

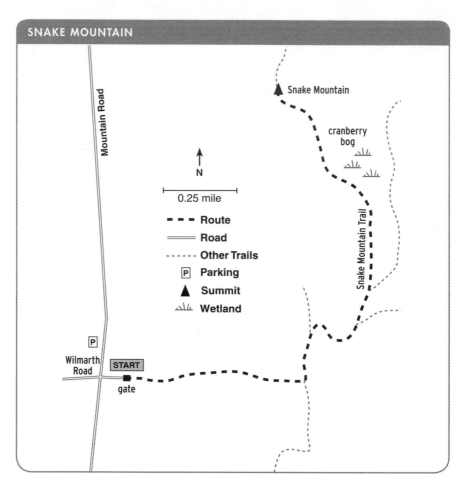

Mountain Road

N

0.25 mile

- - - Route
==== Road
----- Other Trails
P Parking
▲ Summit
⟶ Wetland

Snake Mountain

cranberry
bog

Snake Mountain Trail

P

Wilmarth
Road

START

gate

accommodations and fine dining to travelers. Vacationers could usually take a horse-drawn carriage to their summit accommodations. That's why so many trails in New England are still identified as carriage roads and old bridle paths. Eventually most of these hotels burned to the ground because they were too far away from a source of water to save from fires; today only the foundations remain.

The trail, an old carriage road, starts across from the parking lot through a metal gate. After traveling a half-mile over gradual grades on what used to be a farm hundreds of years ago, the path starts to climb the southern ridge rather quickly. The northern hardwood forest surrounding the route is dotted with hemlock and oak groves. There are several unmarked trail junctions on Snake Mountain. Stick to the most heavily traveled path that will lead to the summit. When in doubt, stay left and head up! Eventually, the path tops out on the ridge and the climbing becomes more gradual and rolling until you reach the summit at 1.8 miles.

Near the summit, there is a lush, moss-covered wetland called Cranberry Bog. We've seen more blueberries here than cranberries. It was created more than 9,000 years ago as the glaciers melted out of New England and is a very sensitive wildlife habitat today.

Keep climbing the ridge until you emerge from the woods to see wide-open skies with stellar views of the surrounding farm country, the high peaks of the Adirondacks, and Lake Champlain. You can even explore the ruins of the foundation of the old Grand View Hotel.

When you need to leave, just head back the way you came.

PLAN B: The nearby Shelburne Orchards offers pick-your-own apples, peaches, grapes, pumpkins, and cherries; cider doughnuts; live music; and the most fun tree rope swing that we have ever tried. The excellent ECHO Lake Aquarium and Science Center in nearby Burlington is a great rainy day option (for directions, see Trip 69). To the south, the alluring Falls of Lana (see Trip 59) and Branbury State Park offer swimming and waterfalls.

NEARBY: You'll find many dining options on US 7 in Shelburne. Burlington a bit farther north has perhaps the widest array of eating opportunities in New England. Middlebury to the south also has excellent options.

Trip 61

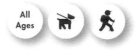

Sunset Ledge

An easy 2.2-mile walk to excellent west-facing views, perfect for a picnic or sunset supper.

Address: Lincoln Gap Road (between Hanks Road and Geary Road North), Lincoln
Difficulty: Easy
Distance: 2.2 miles, round-trip.
Hours: No posted hours
Fee: Free
Contact: Green Mountain National Forest, 802-747-6700, www.fs.usda.gov/greenmountain; Green Mountain Club, 802-244-7037, greenmountainclub.org
Bathrooms: None
Water/Snacks: None
Maps: USGS Lincoln quad
Directions by Car: From the intersection of VT 100 and Lincoln Gap Road in Warren, head west on Lincoln Gap Road for 4.1 miles to the height-of-land and the main parking area (44° 5.682′ N, 72° 55.677′ W). If this is full, you can park at the small auxiliary building you passed on your way.

Few hikes offer such a gorgeous view with such little effort. As the name implies, this rocky outpost has views to the west. Pack dinner and hike in for a gorgeous Vermont sunset or just plan a usual day hike.

From the trailhead, head south on the Long Trail. After an initial steep pitch, you will enter the 25,000-acre Breadloaf Wilderness Area; sign in at the kiosk at the boundary. Wilderness Areas are designated tracts of land set aside by the government where the land and wildlife are free to exist in their natural state, untouched by the hand of humans. You are free to travel through and enjoy these areas, but activities and machinery are limited to keep a pristine wilderness experience.

About halfway up the 1.1-mile hike, you will see an obvious spur path to your left that leads to excellent east-facing views of the Mad River Valley and the Northfield Range, a great spot for a quick breather and a swig of water.

The trail continues on up the spine of the ridge, with patches of sky poking through and occasional views to the east and west. You never feel like you are

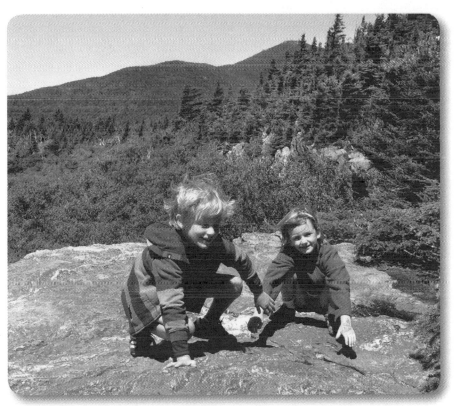

*While a mostly flat hike, the views from the craggy Sunset Ledge are amazing.
(Photo courtesy of Tre McCarney)*

deep in the woods along the path here, and the boreal forest of the ridge tops is great motivation keep moving up to the top. Scramble up and over several rocky ledges, and at 1.1 miles you will finally emerge out onto the wide-open Sunset Ledge with expansive views to the west. With good views comes steep terrain, so keep the kids and pets close here, as there are treacherous drops. Looking to the west, take a glimpse of Lake Champlain and the Adirondacks of New York.

If you are staying in the area or live nearby, pack a meal and try this route in the late afternoon or evening. Bring all the courses, paper plates, and something good to drink—a thermos of hot cocoa is always a hit. (As always, carry out all the trash and food you don't finish.) Watch the twilight hour and sunset, eating your delicious dinner on the ledge. Even though you only have 1.1 miles to hike out afterward, make sure you have headlamps for the hike down.

PLAN B: Head north on the Long Trail for a more challenging hike to Mount Abraham with overnight potential (see Trip 62).

The swimming hole at Bartlett Falls in nearby Bristol will please young and old alike. Its popularity is well founded, as it has something for everyone: a 110-foot-long swimming hole, with shallow and deep water, ledges for jumping, and a waterfall that you can climb behind and even jump through if the current is weak. Come ready to hang out for a few hours, and explore the smaller pools upstream and downstream of this gem. From the trailhead, head west for 7.8 miles to an obvious pullout on Lincoln Gap Road (along the way, the road will be called East River Road, West River Road, and Lincoln Road). The falls are on the left.

NEARBY: The Warren Country Store, a presence in the area since the 1800s when it served as a stagecoach stop, is located in quaint downtown Warren and serves coffee, fresh sandwiches, baked goods, homemade ice cream sandwiches, drinks, and more. Warren and Bristol to its west each have numerous eating options.

There are many huge pieces of land left in the United States that have been made off-limits to roads, machines, and houses. These "wild" places have been set aside just for animals, fish, and plants and for people to come to visit, have adventures, and then leave. These designated Wilderness Areas are typically located on national forest or national park land and have high levels of protection to make sure they remain undeveloped and wild. There are over 109 million acres of officially protected Wilderness Areas in the United States, which is equal to 5 percent of the total land. Humans tend to gradually develop land and build things wherever they can, so Wilderness Areas are places that we've set aside where that won't happen.

Wilderness is officially defined in the Wilderness Act, signed by President Lyndon Johnson in 1964. It states: "A wilderness, in contrast with those areas where man and his own works dominate the landscape, is hereby recognized as an area where the earth and community of life are untrammeled by man, where man himself is a visitor who does not remain." While Wilderness Areas in the western United States may cover millions of acres, most in the Northeast are smaller. The Breadloaf Wilderness in Vermont is 25,000 acres, which is about 30 times the size of Central Park.

In any Wilderness Area, no matter how big or small, certain activities are prohibited to make sure the character of the land is preserved. The most noticeable rules are that there are no roads, no buildings, and no machinery. In this case, "machinery" means anything that uses mechanical advantage; while it may be obvious that a car or bulldozer isn't welcome in a Wilderness, you may not realize that bikes are not allowed either—their gears employ mechanical advantage and they are considered machines. Chainsaws and power tools are also prohibited, so the trail crews must hike in old-fashioned equipment such as 6-foot, 2-person crosscut saws to cut trees out of the trails.

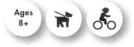

Mount Abraham

A moderate hike up a 4,006-foot peak, complete with crystal clear views, a camping shelter, and a 1970s plane wreck to explore.

Address: Lincoln Gap Road, Lincoln
Distance: 5.2 miles, round-trip
Difficulty: Moderate
Hours: No posted hours
Fee: Free
Contact: Green Mountain National Forest, 802-747-6700 www.fs.usda.gov/
    greenmountain; Green Mountain Club, 802-244-7037, greenmountainclub.org
Bathrooms: None
Water/Snacks: None
Maps: USGS Lincoln quad
Directions by Car: From the intersection of VT 100 and Lincoln Gap Road in
    Warren, head west on Lincoln Gap Road for 4.1 miles to the height-of-land
    and the main parking area (44° 5.682′ N, 72° 55.677′ W). If this is full, you
    can park at the small auxiliary lot you passed on your way.

The hike to Mount Abraham's inspiring panoramic views has a consistently moderate grade, with very few steep sections, making this a great option for young families up for a bit of a challenge. If you can, spend the night on the trail at Battle Shelter. While the trail and shelter are on National Forest property, the shelters in this area are all staffed and managed by the Green Mountain Club (GMC). With an outhouse, dependable water supply, and sheltered camping, Battle Shelter is a great spot for a first family backpacking trip. It can be done as an out-and-back overnight trip, or can be combined with other shelters to the north and south. See GMC's *The Long Trail Guide* for more long-distance backpacking options.

From the parking area, head north along the Long Trail toward Mount Abraham. The trail traverses though mixed hardwood forest to a rest spot between two huge glacial erratic boulders after approximately 0.75 mile (for more about glacial erratics, see Trip 72). Continuing on, the path reaches Battle Shelter at 1.8 miles.

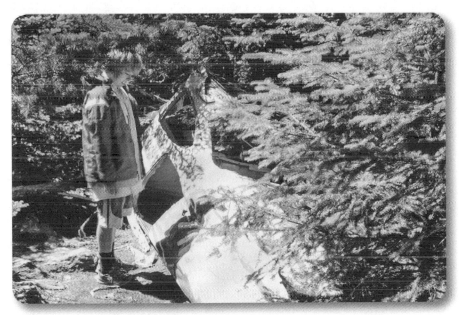

With a little bit of legwork, you can find the wreckage of a plane crash just to the north of the summit of Mount Abraham.

From the shelter, the summit is just 0.8 mile away. This is the steepest section, with many short and fun scrambles up and over granite ledges. The multi-acre summit (2.6 miles) stands at 4,006 feet, making Mount Abraham the fifth highest peak in Vermont. Lake Champlain is to the west; Killington and New Hampshire's Mount Sunapee to the south; Mount Mansfield to the north; and New Hampshire's Presidential Range to the east. This is a fine place to have a picnic, take a nap, and soak in the majestic views.

For the curious, an abandoned plane wreck lies in the woods just beyond the summit. Continue north on the Long Trail for 500 feet. On your left, a well-worn side trail leads into the woods. Follow the side trail for approximately 100 feet to the wreck. According to the GMC caretaker, the two-seater plane went down in bad weather with failing instruments on a stormy day in the mid-1970s. The pilot and passenger survived the crash landing, stumbled out of the plane and found themselves on the Long Trail. Following it south, they hiked themselves out of the woods, leaving the plane behind as proof of their misadventure. Return to the trailhead the way you came (5.2 miles).

PLAN B: Head south from the trailhead for an easier jaunt to Sunset Ledge (see Trip 61). This trip also notes directions for the local favorite, Bartlett Falls (see Trip 61, Plan B).

Warren Falls, perhaps the finest swimming hole in all of Vermont (and maybe New England), exists nearby in Warren. A trip to Mount Abraham would not be complete without a dip in these deep potholes filled with the clear blue-green waters of the Mad River. Ledges for jumping will please the timid and the daring. From the intersection of Lincoln Gap Road and VT 100, head south for 1 mile to a dirt pullout on right. From parking area, follow the trail 100 yards to the right to find the swimming holes.

NEARBY: The Warren Country Store, a presence in the area since the 1800s when it served as a stagecoach stop, is located in quaint downtown Warren and serves coffee, fresh sandwiches, baked goods, homemade ice cream sandwiches, drinks, and more. Warren and Bristol to its west each have numerous eating options.

THE LONG TRAIL

The Long Trail is America's oldest long-distance trail and covers the entire length of Vermont, from Massachusetts to Canada. Following the spine of the Green Mountains, the 273-mile-long path traverses Vermont's highest peaks, as well as swamps, bogs, streams, backcountry lakes, and quaint towns. Each summer, brave souls take this month-long journey. The Long Trail is maintained by the GMC; its excellent *Long Trail Guide* has all the information required to take on this adventure. Many families with kids have taken the plunge and hiked the Long Trail together, and it is also possible to day-hike and do weekend backpack trips on this trail as well. Trips 55, 61, and 62 in this book are all on the Long Trail.

Trip 63

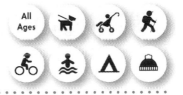

Cross Vermont Bike Trail

This 12.74-mile section of the 90-mile Cross Vermont Trail passes delightful campgrounds and several lakes on its route through peaceful woods.

Address: 2967 Scott Highway (US 302), Groton
Difficulty: Easy–Challenging
Distance: Up to 25.5 miles, round-trip
Hours: No posted hours
Fee: Free
Contact: Cross Vermont Trail Association, 802-498-0079, crossvermont.org
Bathrooms: At the trailhead, Ricker Pond State Park, and Stillwater Campgrounds along the way
Water/Snacks: At the Upper Valley Grill trailhead
Maps: USGS Groton, Knox Mountain, and Marshfield quads; crossvermont.org/images/page_maps/crossvt-map3.pdf
Directions by Car: From the intersection of I-91 and US 302 in Wells River, head west on US 302 for 8.5 miles to the Upper Valley Grill on the left (44° 13.169′ N, 72° 13.418′ W), just before the intersection with VT 232. The building is red and has a single gas pump in front.

Imagine biking on a smooth, old railroad bed through the peaceful farmland and forests of Vermont, swimming in lakes, eating tasty treats, and camping along the way. This is all possible on the Cross Vermont Trail. This multiuse, 90-mile trail crosses the state from Burlington to Wells River following the peaceful grades of the Winooski and Wells river valleys. Much of the trail is situated on old railroad beds with an average grade of under 2 percent, which makes it an excellent path for biking, large-wheeled jogging strollers, and wheelchairs alike. This trip covers one particularly scenic 12.75-mile section of the trail from Groton to Marshfield, but you can bike and camp all the way to Burlington for an epic family adventure! For more information about planning an extended trip, consult the Cross Vermont Trail Association's website.

This route is divided into smaller, bite-sized chunks that you can pick and choose from depending on the abilities of your group. The distances given

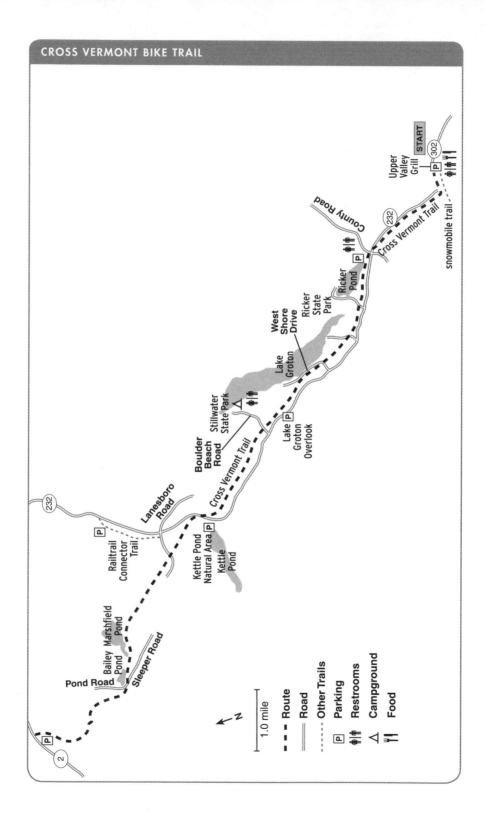

Route
Road
Other Trails
Parking
Restrooms
Campground
Food

1.0 mile

N

Upper Valley Grill

START

302

232

Cross Vermont Trail

snowmobile trail

County Road

Ricker Pond

Ricker State Park

West Shore Drive

Lake Groton

Stillwater State Park

Boulder Beach Road

Cross Vermont Trail

Lake Groton Overlook

Lanesboro Road

232

Railtrail Connector Trail

Kettle Pond Natural Area

Kettle Pond

Bailey Pond

Marshfield Pond

Pond Road

Sleeper Road

2

for each section are one-way. Older kids ages 10 to 12 may want to tackle this 25.5-mile round-trip, which will be a long but rewarding day. Plan to cover fewer sections with younger bikers. We recommend riding hybrid or mountain bikes—the trail is generally smooth, but still a little rough for a road bike with skinny tires.

US 302 to Rickers Mill Trailhead (1.7 miles)
From the Upper Valley Grill parking area, follow the wide shoulder of US 302 for 0.2 mile to Wilson Road on your right. Cross it carefully, then head west on Wilson Road to the railroad bed trail on your right. Follow the railroad bed through ferny hardwood forests to the Rickers Mill trailhead.

Rickers Mill to Kettle Pond (4.5 miles)
This is a beautiful section of trail is highlighted by views of and swimming opportunities at Lake Groton and Kettle Pond—and it may be the best section for young children. At 4.5 miles (just before the bridge over Stillwater Brook), a small spur path leads 400 feet to Kettle Pond, which has great swimming, picnic, and backcountry camping options.

Kettle Pond to Marshfield Village (6.6 miles)
This serene section passes several beautiful ponds and crosses into the Winooski River Watershed. The town of Marshfield makes a good lunch spot before your return trip.

PLAN B: You'll find the Cabot Creamery in nearby Cabot on a winding country road. Factory tours are not all created equal, and this one provides a great mix of getting to see the workings of the massive cheese-making operation with a chance to taste unlimited quantities of Cabot's local cheese.

Easy hikes at Devils Hill (Trip 64) and Big Deer Mountain (Trip 65), and nearby camping make for a great multiday trip.

NEARBY: The Upper Valley Grill at the southern trailhead has a quaint, old-fashioned diner, ice cream stand, and convenience store and deli. Both Marshfield and Groton have many eating options including simple deli sandwiches, pizza, and high-end bistros.

Trip 64

Devils Hill

An easy climb brings you up to open ledges with excellent views over Peacham Bog and Groton State Forest.

Address: Devils Hill Road, Peacham
Difficulty: Easy
Distance: 2.0 miles, round-trip
Hours: No posted hours
Fee: Free
Contact: Groton State Forest, 802-241-3655, vtstateparks.com/pdfs/
groton_trails.pdf; New Discovery State Park, 802-426-3042,
vtstateparks.com/htm/newdiscovery.htm
Bathrooms: None
Water/Snacks: None
Maps: USGS Peacham quad; vtstateparks.com/pdfs/groton_trails.pdf
Directions by Car: From US 302 and Minard Hill Road in Groton Village, head
north on Minard Hill Road, which eventually becomes Peacham Road. After
7.7 miles, turn left on Maple Tree Lane/Town Road 5. In 0.7 mile, turn left on
Green Bay Loop Road. Continue for 1.3 miles and turn right on Devils Hill
Road (just a small sign here; it's just beyond a log home). Proceed to the end
of this narrow dirt lane to the trailhead kiosk and parking area (44° 18.773′ N,
72° 12.799′ W).

This easy hike is perfect when the toddlers are ready to try some hiking on
their own. You will be rewarded with a pleasant walk through the woods on
wide trails to a fine lookout.

Devils Hill lies within the Groton State Forest, a Central Vermont treasure.
There are three campgrounds managed as state parks within the State Forest
boundary: New Discovery, Big Deer, and Stillwater. Chock-full of easy hikes,
ponds and lakes for swimming and paddling, and even a multiuse recreational
path that stretches across Vermont, you can spend a weekend or a week here
exploring all of the nooks and crannies.

From the trailhead, head up Devils Hill Trail, an old road now used for hiking in summer and snowmobiling in winter. The trail is relatively well signed
for the duration, but the equilateral triangles employed by Vermont State Parks

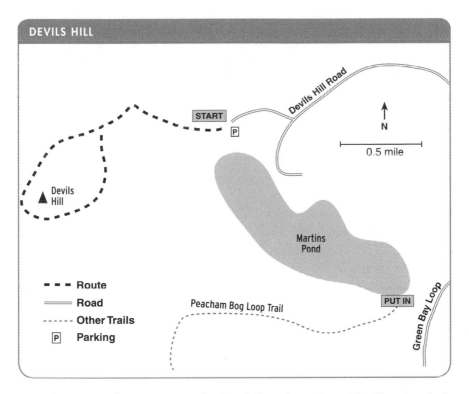

as trail signs confuse some people. Just follow the pointy side. If a triangle is tilted on its side, follow the side with only one corner, rather than two.

The trail soon reaches an intersection (0.25 mile) where you can choose in which direction you want to do the loop. We prefer the counterclockwise direction by far as it leads up the steeper sections and down the more gradual sections, so stay right at the intersection to follow the route as described here.

At 0.9 mile, the trail arrives on the summit of this small but impressive hill. Facing to the west, you can see the entire Groton State Forest with the lovely Peacham Bog sprawling beneath you. If you're visiting in autumn, the colors of the bog are simply incredible. Directly across the valley is Big Deer Mountain (see Trip 65). The summit's open ledges and rock crevices are great for exploration, and the kids will surely want to spend some time here—just keep an eye on the little ones as there are some steep drops in places.

To continue the loop, follow the trail across the crest of the hill and through a lush moss-covered forest. Eventually this old road loops around to the left and reconnects with the trail on which you ascended; turn right here and return to the parking lot.

PLAN B: Nearby Boulder Beach State Park in Groton has an excellent swimming beach that is perfect for a dip after a hike up Devils Hill. Return to US 302 via

Minard Hill Road and take a right. After 1.9 miles, turn right on VT 232. Head north past Ricker Pond State Park to Boulder Beach Road. Turn right here and wind your way through several campgrounds and recreational areas to Boulder Beach. Along the way to Boulder Beach you will pass the Groton Nature Center (on Stillwater Road), which has indoor exhibits, trail information, and special events and concerts throughout summer.

The 90-mile Cross Vermont Bike Trail goes through the Groton State Forest near Devils Hill on a gradual railroad bed. You can easily do some day trips on this section of the trail or take a few days to do the whole thing (see Trip 63).

NEARBY: Groton Village has some fine restaurants and delis for picnic supplies on US 302. Artesano Meadery and Ice Cream makes its signature desserts from local milk and cream, and there even is a see-through beehive in the shop that shows you how bees produce the honey used in Artesano's mead and ice cream.

Trip 65

All Ages $ 🐕 🥾 🏊 ⛺

Big Deer Mountain and Osmore Pond

A perfect 4.1-mile loop hike that leads to the top of a small mountain with great views, hugs the shores of a serene undeveloped pond, and offers backcountry camping options.

Address: New Discovery State Park, VT 232/New Discovery Road, Peacham
Distance: 4.1 miles, round-trip
Difficulty: Easy
Hours: 10 A.M. to sunset, Memorial Day weekend to Columbus Day
Fee: $3 children 14 and older, $2 children ages 4–13
Contact: New Discovery State Park, 802-426-3042, vtstateparks.com/htm/newdiscovery.htm
Bathrooms: At New Discovery Campground and Osmore Pond Day Use Area
Water/Snacks: At New Discovery Campground and Osmore Pond Day Use Area
Maps: USGS Marshfield quad; vtstateparks.com/pdfs/groton_trails.pdf
Directions by Car: From US 302 and VT 232 in Groton Village, head north on VT 232 for 9.3 miles to New Discovery State Park on your right. If the campground is open, park near the equestrian campsites. Head past the entrance booth, straight down the campground road for several hundred yards to a clearing where the road branches off to the left. The equestrian campsites are located at this intersection (44° 19.175′ N, 72° 17.243′ W). Ask park staff at the gate the best place to leave your car. If the campground is closed, just park outside the gate and walk to the equestrian campsites with the hitching posts.

The grades of Big Deer Mountain Trail are mellow and the kids will love the great views from the summit and the chance to go for a dip in Osmore Pond. The trail is mostly flat or gradual, with short uphill bursts near the top. This fun loop hike lies within Groton State Forest, which is home to a number of easy hikes, ponds, and lakes, and sections of the Cross Vermont Bike Trail. The campground where you begin is just one of three campgrounds managed as state parks within Groton State Forest. You can turn your visit into an overnight trip by staying at New Discovery or by backcountry camping on Osmore Pond and Kettle Pond, to which you can either hike or paddle.

From campsite 45 in the New Discovery Campground, proceed past the gate to a narrow, flat, woods road. After 0.3 mile, the road reaches Big Deer

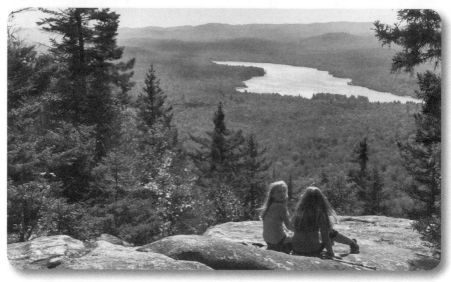

Warm up on the sunny granite slabs of Big Deer Mountain.

Mountain Trail in a stand of red pine. Turn right here and proceed for 1.1 miles through beautiful hardwood forests and easy grades. The trail passes a decaying lean-to from the Civilian Conservation Corps era. The footpath starts to climb gradually, and 0.25 mile before the summit it comes to a trail intersection. Stay to the left here and continue on up the short pitch to the top of Big Deer Mountain with nice open ledges and great views to the south and west (1.7 miles).

To complete the loop, head back down to the intersection below the summit (1.9 miles) and turn left. Continue on this trail for 0.9 mile (past Hosmer Brook Trail on the left) to Osmore Pond Trail. Turn right and head north along the shores of Osmore Pond (3.0 miles) and past three lovely backcountry campsites to which you can paddle or hike. Continue on Osmore Pond trail across a forest road to return to the New Discovery Campground (4.1 miles).

PLAN B: Stop for a swim at nearby Boulder Beach State Park in Groton. Head south for 4 miles on VT 232 and make a sharp left on Boulder Beach Road. Wind your way through several campgrounds and recreational areas to Boulder Beach. The Groton Nature Center on Stillwater Road has indoor exhibits, trail information, and special events and concerts throughout summer.

A section of the 90-mile Cross Vermont Bike Trail cuts through Groton State Forest near Big Deer on a gradual railroad bed (see Trip 63).

NEARBY: Groton Village has some fine restaurants and delis for picnic supplies on US 302. See Trip 64 for more on the local Artesano Meadery and Ice Cream.

Section 7

Northern Vermont

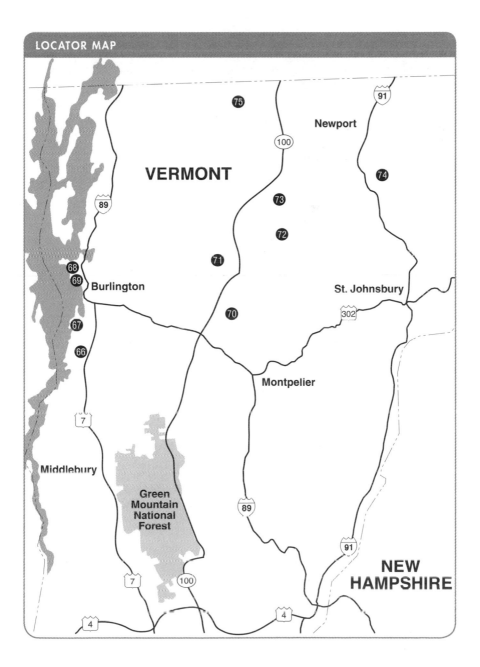

LOCATOR MAP

91

75

Newport

100

VERMONT

74

89

73

72

71

68
69
Burlington

St. Johnsbury

70

302

67

66

Montpelier

7

Middlebury

Green
Mountain
National
Forest

89

91

NEW
HAMPSHIRE

7

100

4

4

Trip 66

All Ages | $ | 🐕 | 🚶 | ⛄

Mount Philo

An easy climb up this small but prominent mountain rewards you with commanding views of the Adirondack and Green mountains, and grassy picnic areas overlooking pastoral valleys.

Address: 5425 Mount Philo Road, Charlotte
Difficulty: Easy
Distance: 2.4 miles, round-trip
Hours: 10 A.M. to sunset
Fee: $3 adults, $2 children ages 4–14
Contact: Mount Philo State Park, 802-425-2390 (office), 888-409-7579 (reservations), vtstateparks.com/htm/philo.htm
Bathrooms: At trailhead and summit
Water/Snacks: Water at summit and campground
Maps: USGS Mount Philo quad; vtstateparks.com/pdfs/philo.pdf
Directions by Car: From the intersection of I-89 and US 7 in Burlington, head south on US 7 for 4.6 miles to Falls Road in Shelburne; take a left. Follow Falls Road for 7.2 miles; along the way it becomes Mount Philo Road. Turn left onto State Park Road. Parking for House Rock trailhead is on your left (44° 16.698′ N, 73° 13.347′ W).

Mount Philo State Park is a jewel, with well-maintained trails, a small but quiet campground, and a plethora of Civilian Conservation Corps-era buildings. But the highlight is the commanding views from the summit of this small mountain. Even though it sits squarely in the middle of pastoral farm country, Mount Philo rises abruptly from the surrounding fields and pastures to gain stellar views of Lake Champlain, the Adirondacks, and the Green Mountains. A road leads to the summit, so on weekends it can get busy, but it is still very much worth the trip. Weekdays are much quieter, and late fall and early spring are excellent times to visit.

From House Rock trailhead, head uphill through a forest dominated by sugar maples. Some nice rock stairs lead to the large glacial erratic boulder from which the trail gets its name—it's as big as house! A massive sheet of ice carried this giant boulder thousands of years ago and deposited it on this hillside like nothing more than a piece of gravel.

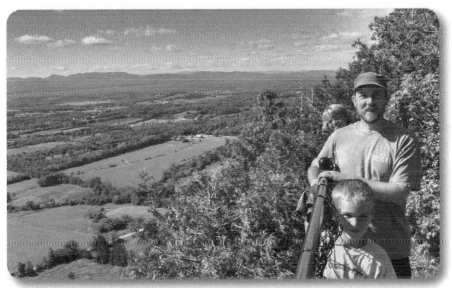
Mount Philo rises above the surrounding farmland to provide a magnificent view of the patchwork fields, Lake Champlain, and the Green Mountains.

Continue on the trail after it crosses a road at 0.3 mile. Many large trees make this section of the route a great spot for playing hide-and-seek on the go. When you reach the Devils Chair Trail a few hundred yards beyond, stay to the left and proceed straight to the summit (0.6 mile). From the open summit, look for the excellent viewpoints on the right to Lake Champlain and the Adirondacks. The summit's grassy lawn offers Adirondack chairs and a picnic pavilion that can be rented for large groups. Many other, more secluded picnic areas are sprinkled around the summit, each complete with a picnic table and a fire ring.

To descend, continue on past the parking lot at the summit, staying to the right on Old Carriage Road along the top of the cliffs. Take a right when you reach the auto road again. This road is one-way and you will be walking down facing any cars coming up from below. After 0.2 mile, the road reaches Devils Chair Trail on the right. Follow this trail along the base of the cliffs to its intersection with House Rock Trail (1.5 miles). Head downhill, cross the road again, and follow House Rock Trail back to the parking lot.

To extend the fun, book a campsite in the very small and rustic campground nestled on the side of the mountain. Trails lead directly to the summit from the campground. In winter, the park road becomes one of the most exciting sledding hills in New England!

PLAN B: The nearby Shelburne Orchards offers pick-your-own apples, peaches, grapes, pumpkins, and cherries; cider doughnuts; live music; and the most fun tree rope swing that we have ever tried. Standing on a steep hillside, you swing out over the abyss and brush the leaves of the apple trees beyond.

The excellent ECHO Lake Aquarium and Science Center in nearby Burlington is a great rainy day option (for directions, see Trip 69).

NEARBY: Many dining options exist on US 7 in Shelburne, and Burlington a bit farther north has perhaps the widest array of eating opportunities in New England.

Trip 67

Shelburne Farms

Easy paths meander through farmland, meadows, and hills that give magnificent views of the Lake Champlain shoreline and surrounding farmland and mountains.

Address: 1611 Harbor Road, Shelburne
Difficulty: Easy–Moderate
Distance: 1.0–4.5 miles, round-trip
Hours: 9 A.M. to 5 P.M., May–October
Fee: $8 adults, $5 kids 3–17
Contact: Shelburne Farms, shelburnefarms.org
Bathrooms: At Welcome Center and Farm Barn
Water/Snacks: Water, snacks, sandwiches, and picnic fare are available at the
    Farm Barn and the food truck snack bar
Maps: USGS Juniper Island quad; shelburnefarms.org/visit/walking-trails
Directions by Car: From the intersection of I-189 and US 7 in South Burlington,
    head south on US 7 for 2.9 miles. In Shelburne, veer right onto Bay Road and
    continue for 1.7 miles to the Shelburne Farms parking lot (44° 23.738′ N,
    73° 14.827′ W).

Shelburne Farms is the quintessential family outing in Vermont. With great hiking, expansive views, an educational farm, petting area, cheese making facility, Lake Champlain shoreline, and nearby nature trails and apple orchards, it is simply a great place to spend time with kids. There is a lot to see and do, so allow for a full day or more. (Note: Dogs are allowed November 1–March 31.)

Originally designed by Frederick Law Olmsted (who also designed New York's Central Park and Boston's Emerald Necklace), the farm is a testament to landscape design and straddles an interesting mix of natural and man-made landscapes. Almost every vista, pasture, and forest has been thought out and designed to allow for maximum functionality and beauty.

The best way to see the property is on Farm Trail. Starting at the Welcome Center and parking area, take a tractor-drawn shuttle to the Farm Barn, where you'll find the trailhead as well as a children's farmyard, a cheese making shop, a food cart, and the headquarters for the farm's educational programs and

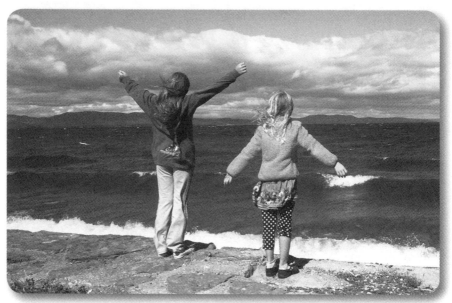

Lake Champlain on a windy day can be an exciting place!

camps. Since the trail begins and ends here, there's no need to soak it all in at once.

From the Farm Barn trailhead, take Farm Trail loop counterclockwise up the hill past the Sheep's Knoll. This open hillside presents excellent opportunities for log-rolling down the hill. Try a relay race of running up the hill and rolling down it! Continuing on counterclockwise, you will hike through the woods past the market garden on the right, a great place to stop and view the prolific gardens tended by the staff and volunteers.

After turning left and right, the path crosses through open pasture down the beautiful shoreline of Lake Champlain. This is a great picnic spot and the halfway point in your walk. Continue on the route through open pasture and woods, then on to the appropriately named Whimsy Meadow, full of wildflowers, a maze of paths through the flowers and high grasses, shade trees, and probably some fairies and gnomes as well.

Continuing on around the loop, the high point of the property, Lone Tree Hill, awaits with excellent views of Lake Champlain, the Adirondacks to the west, and the rolling Green Mountains to the east. Descend Lone Tree Hill to return to the massive Farm Barn.

If you are short on time or the kids aren't up for a long hike, you can take the 0.5-mile Lone Tree Hill Trail to the high point to catch the view.

PLAN B: There is much to do in the area, so you can plan to pack your day very full. The nearby Shelburne Orchards offers pick-your-own apples, peaches, grapes, pumpkins, and cherries; cider doughnuts; live music; and the most fun tree rope swing that we have ever tried. Standing on a steep hillside, you swing out over the abyss and brush the leaves of the apple trees beyond. A thrilling ride! The excellent ECHO Lake Aquarium and Science Center in nearby Burlington is a great rainy day option (for directions, see Trip 69).

NEARBY: Burlington has perhaps the widest array of eating opportunities in New England. From trendy food carts to high-end cuisine, it has something for everyone. For the most options, head to Church Street, a pedestrian-only stretch of restaurants, shops, and music venues. The kids will have a blast sampling tasty treats from the food vendors and watching the many street performers and musicians.

Trip 68

Ages 8+

Burlington's Intervale

Take a pastoral ride on dirt roads and bike paths, past farms and along the Winooski River—all right in the heart of Vermont's largest city.

Address: Intervale Center, 180 Intervale Road, Burlington
Distance: 8.0–10.0 miles, biking
Difficulty: Moderate
Hours: No posted hours
Fee: Free
Contact: Local Motion, 802-861-2700, localmotion.org; Burlington Parks and Recreation, 802-864-0123, enjoyburlington.com/parks/bikepath1.cfm
Bathrooms: At Intervale Center
Water/Snacks: At Intervale Center
Maps: USGS Burlington and Colchester quads; localmotion.org/images/documents/fullguide.pdf
Directions by Car: From I-89, Exit 14 W, take US 2 west. Follow US 2 for 1.2 miles. Turn right on South Prospect Street. Continue for 0.3 mile, then turn left onto Colchester Street, then make an immediate right onto North Prospect Street. Follow this for 0.9 mile; as you cross Riverside Avenue at 0.6 mile, this street becomes Intervale Road. Intervale Center will be on your right; just as the road turns to gravel, there is a large public parking area, also on your right (44° 29.578′ N, 73° 12.332′ W).

You may never have imagined that you could bike through peaceful river valley farmland, along the banks of a lazily winding river, through flood-plain forests and up to a stone castle viewing tower—all in Burlington. The trip described here is actually a shortened, 8.0-mile version of the excellent 10.1-mile Cycle the City loop, jointly developed by the City of Burlington and Local Motion, a nonprofit human-powered transportation advocacy group. The 8.0-mile trip described here is 100 percent bike paths and gravel roads, whereas the official loop includes some street biking and is a couple miles longer. If your family is up for the challenge, we highly recommend the full 10.1-mile loop as well. More information and a map of the full loop is available at localmotion.org/images/documents/fullguide.pdf.

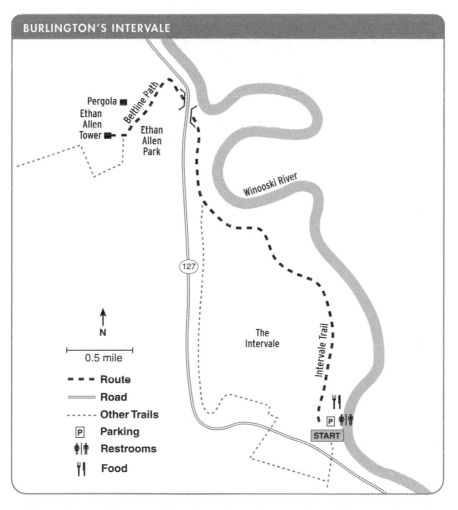

Pergola ■
Ethan
Allen
Tower ■
Ethan
Allen
Park

Beltline Path

Winooski River

127

The
Intervale

Intervale Trail

N

0.5 mile

■ ■ ■ Route
Road
Other Trails
P Parking
Restrooms
Food

START

From the parking area, head north on the gravel road known from this point northward as Intervale Trail. Burlington's Intervale is technically undevelopable for building because of its low-lying, flood-prone land, so it is now a 3,900-acre reserve that is protected as conservation and farm lands. This land has been farmed for thousands of years by native people and by settlers, and today you can bike along the gravel road and see the many small-scale and organic farmers that now call this place home. Hop off your bikes to explore, meet some of the farmers/entrepreneurs, and take a stroll through the huge community gardens.

After 1.0 mile, the trail meets a large open field and the road splits. Take the left-hand fork and continue around the field and then along the banks of the Winooski River. This slow moving section of river makes for good swimming or fishing.

From the river, continue on the dirt road and follow the signs to the Ethan Allen Homestead. The small farmhouse at the Ethan Allen Homestead was the Revolutionary War hero's home for his last years of life, and now serves as a memorial to his life. Inquire at the gift shop about tours.

From the homestead, follow the paved Beltline bike path north for 0.5 mile to a bridge over VT 127. After the bridge, the path enters Ethan Allen Park. Follow the paved bike path for 500 feet to an intersection. Stay left here and follow the gently rolling path for another 0.3 mile to a T intersection; make another left. Follow this path for 0.25 mile to your halfway point: the Ethan Allen Tower.

Lock your bikes to a tree, then head up the very short path to an open ridge with great views of Burlington. On top of the ridge is a 50-foot-high stone tower, complete with turrets and arrow slits, built in 1905 as a memorial to Ethan Allen (open weekends Mother's Day to Memorial Day, open daily Memorial Day to Columbus Day). Climb the stairs to see the panoramic views of the farm, the Winooski River, and the city. Have a picnic on the ridge, then head back the way you came for a round-trip of 8.0 miles.

PLAN B: The ECHO Lake Aquarium and Science Center is a great rainy day option. One of the only freshwater aquariums in the country, it has a wide variety of hands-on exhibits. Also, several ferry sightseeing tour operators offering day and dinner cruises can be found on the waterfront (for directions, see Trip 69). One inexpensive option to just see the lake from the deck of a boat is to take the Burlington–Port Kent, New York, ferry that leaves from the King Street Dock a couple blocks away.

NEARBY: Burlington has perhaps the widest array of eating opportunities in New England. It has something for everyone, including trendy food carts, pizza, Asian food, and high-end cuisine. For the most options, head to Church Street, a pedestrian-only stretch of restaurants, shops, and music venues. The kids will have a blast sampling tasty treats from the food vendors and watching the many street performers and musicians.

Trip 69

Ages 8+

Island Line Bike Trail

Bike from the urban core of Burlington past peaceful wooded shoreline to the grand causeways that cross Lake Champlain—all on level-graded, dedicated bike paths!

Address: ECHO Lake Aquarium and Science Center, 1 College Street, Burlington
Difficulty: Easy–Challenging
Distance: 4.0–38.0 miles round-trip
Hours: No posted hours for trail; contact Local Motion for current bike ferry schedule
Fee: Free for day use; contact Local Motion for current bike ferry fees
Contact: Burlington Parks and Recreation, 802-864-0123, enjoyburlington.com/parks/bikepath1.cfm; Local Motion, 802-861-2700, localmotion.org
Bathrooms: At Local Motion Bike Shop, North Beach Campground, Leddy Park
Water/Snacks: At Local Motion Bike Shop, North Beach Campground, Leddy Park
Maps: USGS Burlington, Colchester, and Colchester Point quads; localmotion.org/programs/islandline/trail
Directions by Car: From I-89, Exit 14 W, take US 2/Main Street west. Continue on US 2/Main Street for 2.2 miles. When Main Street takes a hard right turn and becomes Lake Street, follow it to College Street. The ECHO Lake Aquarium and Science Center (ECHO) will be on your left (44° 28.607′ N, 73° 13.217′ W). Park anywhere near here and proceed toward the waterfront to the obvious bike path. Local Motion Bike Shop, the trailhead for this route, is just to the south of ECHO on the path.

This delightful bike trip has so many highlights: a flat, easy grade for the duration, a beautiful wooded shoreline ride, interesting stops and beaches along the way, a giant causeway that slices through Lake Champlain, and a bike ferry connecting sections of the causeway. The path is paved for most of the way, and the causeway is fine-packed stone dust. Any type of bike will be able to make the trip, and even the youngest bikers will have a great time on shorter sections. There is some street cycling on this route, but all street sections of the Island Line Trail south of Grand Isle are on quiet residential streets, are marked clearly, and have separate lanes for bikes; north of Grand Isle some

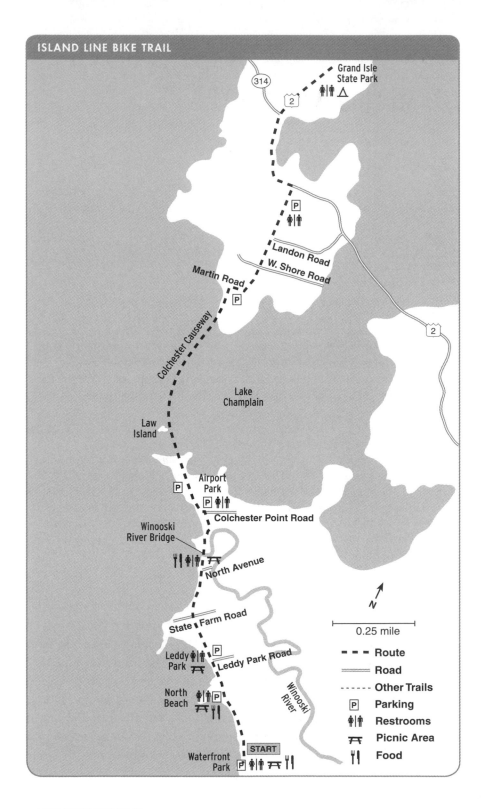

Grand Isle
State Park

314
2

Landon Road
W. Shore Road

Martin Road

Colchester Causeway

Lake
Champlain

2

Law
Island

Airport
Park

Colchester Point Road

Winooski
River Bridge

North Avenue

State Farm Road

Leddy
Park

Leddy Park Road

Winooski
River

North
Beach

START

Waterfront
Park

N

0.25 mile

- - - Route
=== Road
----- Other Trails
P   Parking
👫 Restrooms
🪑 Picnic Area
🍴 Food

sections are along a state highway with a shoulder and are recommended only for older or more experienced bikers.

As described, this south–north route begins near ECHO along the Burlington waterfront and heads north. If you want a shorter trip, there are many parks along the lake to the north that make ideal starting points if you'd like to arrange a shuttle. Each section of the trail is described below, so just pick what works for you and set off. Remember that the distances are listed one-way. All of the starting and ending points listed below have parking and access to the trail.

Local Motion to North Beach Campground (1.9 miles)

Local Motion—a Burlington-based, nonprofit bike and pedestrian advocacy organization—has a bike shop along the Burlington waterfront. It has bike rentals, drinks, snacks, and maps and makes an excellent starting point for a bike trip. This flat and easy section passes by the inline skating rink (converted to an outdoor ice rink in winter) and the Burlington Skate Park as it makes its way north to North Beach. This is a lovely urban beach with sunbathing and swimming, but its municipal campground, a rarity in New England, really sets it apart.

North Beach Campground to Airport Park (4.5 miles)

This section becomes more wooded and quiet as it follows the Lake Champlain shoreline and passes several beaches, all worth exploring. Along the way, the fantastic Leddy Park hosts an indoor ice arena, as well as a great swimming beach loaded with driftwood. Hours can be spent beachcombing, playing in driftwood forts or swimming along this section. Leddy Park also has parking and restrooms. Stop by the Auer Family Boathouse, otherwise known as "Charlie's" (located just to the south of the Winooski River Bridge) to enjoy a serene park-like setting on the water, ultra low-cost boat rentals, and a small snack bar. Play in the swings and pet the friendly dogs before heading back on the trail.

After crossing the bridge, the trail goes through more woodland and then follows city streets for several blocks before arriving at Airport Park.

Airport Park to Grand Isle (4.7 miles)

This is the most majestic and distinctive section of the trail. Not only will you ride your bikes on an elevated causeway through the middle of America's sixth largest lake, but you also have the unique pleasure of taking a bike ferry that connects two sections of causeway. (The causeway is open year-round, but the bike ferry operates Friday through Sunday, mid-June through Labor

Day, then weekends-only through Columbus Day. Check localmotion.org for schedule updates).

From Airport Park, the Island Line Bike Trail heads north through dense woods before emerging onto the raised causeway that crosses Lake Champlain to Grand Isle. Originally built for trains, this causeway has been retrofitted with firm stonedust and restricted to bikers and walkers. The path crosses a bridge (a great spot for some jumping and swimming), and soon reaches the bike ferry which will deliver you to the southern tip of Grand Isle. If the bike ferry is closed, this is still a worthwhile section to bike.

North End of Causeway to Grand Isle State Park (8.1 miles)

This section is for older or more experienced bikers as it does involve a mix of biking on bike paths, quiet rural roads, and busier state highways with shoulders. Getting to Grand Isle State Park is fantastic though, and the park makes for an amazing bike camping destination if your family is up for it. Getting here from downtown Burlington means a 19-mile day on loaded bikes, but you will be rewarded with a peaceful campground on the shore of the lake, beautiful campsites and lean-tos to rent, and a perfect introduction to the world of bike camping. Nothing beats marshmallows by the fire along the lakeshore after a day of biking and the satisfaction of knowing you got there under your own power! Be sure to take the bike ferry schedule into account when planning your camping trip.

PLAN B: The ECHO Lake Aquarium and Science Center near the trailhead is a great rainy day option (for directions, see Trip 69). One of the only freshwater aquariums in the country, it has a wide variety of hands-on exhibits. Also at the waterfront near ECHO there are several ferry sightseeing tours operators offering day and dinner cruises. A cheap option to just see the lake from the perspective of a boat is to take the Burlington–Port Kent, New York, ferry that leaves from the King Street Dock a couple blocks away.

NEARBY: Burlington has perhaps the widest array of eating opportunities in Vermont. There is something for everyone, including trendy food carts, pizza, Asian food and high-end cuisine. For the most options, head to Church Street, a pedestrian-only stretch of restaurants, shops, and music venues. The kids will have a blast sampling tasty treats from the food vendors and watching the many street performers and musicians.

Trip 70

Ages 8+

Mount Hunger

This strenuous hike on a wet trail is best for more experienced hikers, and it leads to amazing views on the bald summit.

Address: Sweet Farm Road, Waterbury
Difficulty: Challenging
Distance: 4.0 miles, round-trip
Hours: No posted hours
Fee: Free
Contact: Green Mountain Club, 802-244-7037, greenmountainclub.org
Bathrooms: None
Water/Snacks: None
Maps: USGS Stowe quad; *Mount Mansfield and the Worcester Range Hiking Trail Map* (Green Mountain Club)
Directions by Car: From I-89, Exit 10 in Waterbury, head north on VT 100 past Ben & Jerry's Ice Cream. In 1.1 miles take your first right at Guptil Road. Proceed for 2.0 miles, take a right on Maple Street, and immediately turn right onto Loomis Hill Road, which eventually becomes Sweet Farm Road. Continue 2.5 miles to the signed trailhead parking area on your right (44° 24.158′ N, 72° 40.539′ W).

Mount Hunger's prominence over the nearby landscape and its bald summit make this more difficult trip well worth the effort for children over 8. Though it's just over 2.0 miles one-way, we've seen many crying 4-year-olds on this trail; your older, more aggressive hikers, however, will get a great sense of accomplishment from this short yet challenging hike. Combined with nearby swimming holes in Stowe or Bolton, this can make for a positively great day. Also: bring some bug spray if visiting in June or July; the blackflies on the summit at that time of year can send you scurrying back down the trail.

The defining characteristic of this trail is unrelenting steepness. The first few hundred yards from the trailhead are rooty, then the trail starts up at a steep grade and doesn't really stop until it pops out on the summit. About a third of the way up, the path crosses two small tributary streams, and at about the 1.0-mile mark it passes an impressive, unnamed, little waterfall. No

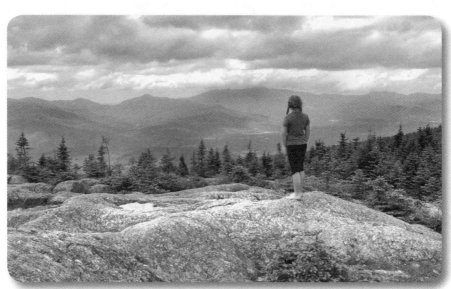

After a steep hike up through the woods, the summit of Mount Hunger is an oasis of open skies and panoramic vistas.

swimming holes here, but there is a pool deep enough to dip your head in on a hot day.

Next come the ledges. The second mile is punctuated by short sections of ledgy terrain with scrambles. These can be great fun for the kids—just keep them close and spot each other on the steep sections.

About a 0.1 mile from the summit, the trail to the equally exciting White Rock Mountain heads off to the right. Continue straight, over ledges and boulders, to finally reach one of the best views in this part of the state (2.0 miles). Situated at the southern end of Vermont's Worcester Range, Mount Hunger is actually in the same range as Elmore Mountain (see Trip 72) as well as White Rock Mountain, Stowe Pinnacle, and Worcester Mountain. Mount Hunger is the tallest of the mountains in this small yet impressive range, and the view from the summit extends from Mount Mansfield directly across the valley to the west, and to New Hampshire's Presidentials to the east.

Return along the same route.

PLAN B: Your kids may mutiny if you make it all the way here without a stop at the Ben & Jerry's factory on VT 100 in nearby Waterbury. Factory tours, free samples, and a full ice cream shop will delight. For a great after-ice-cream swim, head to nearby Bolton Potholes. Several deep potholes and a wide and shallow sandy bottomed pool make this a great spot on a summer day. You won't be the only ones there, but it is still a refreshing and fun place. From Ben & Jerry's, head south on VT 100 to US 2, turn right and drive 6.7 miles to the elementary school in Bolton. The swimming hole is directly behind the school. Nearby Bingham Falls and Moss Glen Falls (both in Stowe) are great short hikes to some of the most beautiful waterfalls in the state.

NEARBY: Stowe Village is chock-full of cafés, bagel shops, pizza places, and delis. Waterbury also has many fine places to grab a bite.

When the temperature drops and the snow begins to fall, it's tempting to shelve the outdoor guidebooks, hang up the backpacks, put away the boots, and resign your family to months of indoor board games by the fire. But it isn't long before cabin fever strikes. "I'm bored!" whine the kids. Fortunately, with a little planning and a robust spirit of adventure, it's easy to get outside and enjoy the winter wonderland that makes northern New England a top destination for outdoor enthusiasts around the world. Here are a few trips your family will enjoy even in winter:

- **Gilsland Farm, ME (Trip 7):** Rent snowshoes or bring your own cross-country skis and hit the trails at Maine Audubon's headquarters, which offers hundreds of public programs with staff naturalists on hand, such as winter carnival where you can help construct a snow fort (snow permitting, of course)!

- **Bear Brook State Park, NH (Trip 46):** The cross-country ski trail network in New Hampshire's second largest state park is not to be missed. Gentle, rolling terrain leads through forests of massive white pines to frozen ponds. Broken Boulder, Pitch Pine, and Bobcat trails are all recommended for families.

- **Merck Forest and Farmland Center, VT (Trip 56):** At this working farm and forest, winter wonderland is in full effect, sleigh rides and all. Consider a moonlight cross-country ski or snowshoe through farm fields on Burke Trail or reserve one of the popular backcountry cabins for a truly memorable winter adventure.

- **Mount Philo, VT (Trip 66):** A Burlington-area winter destination for many, Mount Philo has some of the best sledding in Vermont on the unplowed park road up the mountain. If you want to "earn your turns," consider showshoeing to the summit from House Rock Trailhead, taking in the spectacular views at the top, and then sledding down the park road.

Whether you're heading to one of the above destinations or keeping closer to home, winter adventuring is more fun when you incorporate activities such as constructing snow sculptures and forts, searching for animal tracks, throwing snowballs, and making snow angels.

Trip 71

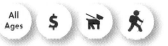

Mount Mansfield Ridge

After an easy drive, this ridge-top trail winds through alpine tundra to the highest point in Vermont for breathtaking views—all for minimal effort.

Address: Toll Road, Stowe
Difficulty: Easy
Distance: 2.4 miles, round-trip
Hours: No posted hours, Memorial Day weekend–October 19
Fee: Contact Stowe Mountain Resort for current Auto Toll Road fees
Contact: Underhill State Park, 802-899-3022, vtstateparks.com/htm/underhill. htm; Stowe Mountain Resort (Auto Toll Road information), 888-253-4849 (toll-free), 802-253-3000, stowe.com/activities/summer/auto-toll-road
Bathrooms: At base area and summit station
Water/Snacks: At base area and summit station
Maps: USGS Mount Mansfield quad; *Mount Mansfield and the Worcester Range Hiking Trail Map* (Green Mountain Club)
Directions by Car: From the intersection of VT 100 and VT 108 in Stowe, head north on VT 108 toward Stowe Mountain Resort for 5.8 miles to the Auto Toll Road entrance on the left (44° 30.643′ N, 72° 45.948′ W).

Unlike most of the trips in this book, which depend 100 percent on human power to get to the final destination, this option gives people of all abilities the chance to experience the alpine splendor of Vermont's highest peak.

Driving the historic Auto Toll Road does require a hefty toll; check with Stowe Mountain Resort for current prices. While parking at a trailhead at the bottom of a mountain is usually far less expensive if not free, paying the toll to get up the road has its advantages and may be the only way some families will be able to experience this part of the world. Driving the road is an exhilarating experience in itself, as it winds its way up the steep flanks of Mount Mansfield. Once the car reaches the summit station, your 2.4-mile round-trip hike is completely above treeline. The car does all of the heavy lifting; your family gets to just soak it up and enjoy it.

If you view the mountain's profile from the east or the west, the summit ridge resembles an elongated facial profile, with a distinct forehead, nose,

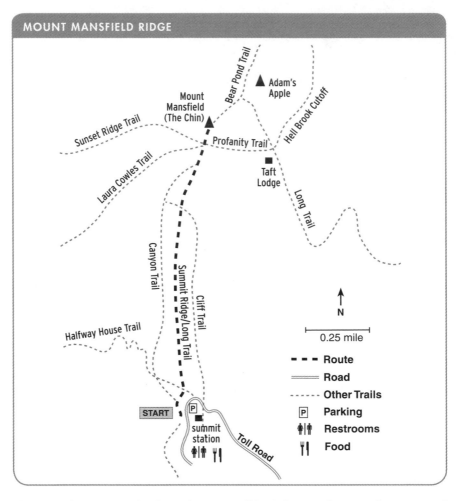

Bear Pond Trail

▲ Adam's Apple

Mount Mansfield (The Chin)

Sunset Ridge Trail

Profanity Trail

Hell Brook Cutoff

Laura Cowles Trail

■ Taft Lodge

Long Trail

Canyon Trail

Summit Ridge/Long Trail

Cliff Trail

N

0.25 mile

Halfway House Trail

- - - Route

═══ Road

- - - Other Trails

P Parking

†|† Restrooms

†† Food

START

P

summit station

†|† ††

Toll Road

chin—and even an Adam's apple. You will be hiking right over the Nose and up to the Chin, the highest point on the mountain at 4,393 feet. Your overall elevation gain and drop is just 500 feet; this route requires surprisingly little effort to get to such an exposed and beautiful place.

From the summit station near the Nose, park and head north on Summit Ridge Trail (part of the Long Trail that goes the entire length of the state) toward the Chin.

The hike along this exposed ridge takes you through hundreds of acres of alpine tundra, an ecosystem that is very rare in New England. Vermont only has three peaks that harbor this ecosystem (Camels Hump, Mount Abraham, and Mount Mansfield). It is characterized by a complete lack of trees, and very limited plant growth. Because the conditions are so harsh in alpine zones with wind, ice, and cold temperatures, it takes hundreds of years for soils to form from eroded rocks, and then hundreds more for grasses and sedges to take root. Wildflowers, lichens, and low shrubs may form as well. Given how long it takes vegetation to establish itself in tundra landscapes, it is very important that all hikers—no matter how small—stick to the established trails so as not to disturb this very fragile environment.

The treeless ridge treats you to wide-open expansive views for the entire hike, so take your time and soak it in. The summit at the Chin provides 360-degree views of Vermont, New Hampshire, New York, and Lake Champlain. The landscape is simply astounding.

For adventurous souls who travel above treeline for extended periods, properly prepare yourself and your family with warm layers, wind protection, and rain gear. Weather can change quickly here and the effects can be dangerous and devastating. Each year, hundreds of hikers in alpine zones get hypothermia in summer months due to being unprepared for storms, rain, and high winds on these exposed ridges. Keep an eye out for lightning storms and retreat quickly if you see lightning anywhere in the vicinity, as exposed ridge tops are the last place you want to be in a lightning storm.

PLAN B: Bingham Falls is just up VT 108 from the Toll Road. A 0.25-mile hike leads to stunning waterfalls with some shallow swimmable holes below the main fall. Expect big crowds here, but it's a beautiful spot nonetheless.

You'll also find excellent swimming at Fosters, a deep pool in the West Branch Little River on Notchbrook Road, 0.25 mile from VT 108. The pool is chock-full of brook trout, and you can try to catch them with your hands where they hide behind the falls.

There is plenty of camping available at Underhill State Park and Smugglers' Notch State Park.

NEARBY: Stowe Village is home to many cafés, bagel shops, pizza places, and delis.

Trip 72

Ages 5+ $ 🐕   🚶   🏊   ⛺

Elmore Mountain

Hike this moderate ridge-top loop to a fire tower with open ledge views, boulder caves to explore, and a balancing rock.

Address: Elmore State Park, 856 VT 12, Lake Elmore
Difficulty: Moderate
Distance: 3.2-mile loop or 2.5 miles, out-and-back round-trip
Hours: 9 A.M. to sunset, Memorial Day weekend–Columbus Day weekend
Fee: $3 adults, $2 children ages 4–14
Contact: Elmore State Park, 802-888-2982, vtstateparks.com/htm/elmore.htm
Bathrooms: Available at Bath House
Water/Snacks: Available at Bath House
Maps: USGS Morrisville quad; vtstateparks.com/pdfs/elmore.pdf
Directions by Car: From intersection of VT 100 and VT 12 in Morrisville, head east on VT 12 for 3.6 miles. An obvious sign for Elmore State Park will be on your right. Check in at the ranger station. Proceed past the campground (on right); follow the road as it switchbacks up the ridge to the trailhead parking and gate (44° 32.648′ N, 72° 31.694′ W).

The trails to Elmore Mountain have been upgraded into a fun 3.2-mile loop, with ledgy views and a five-story fire tower to climb! While hikers of most ages will enjoy the trail, parents with toddlers may find reaching the summit a challenge as there are steep, wet sections of trail and because the fire tower has very few safety railings. This trip describes a clockwise route up the steeper, wetter sections and down the more gradual sections.

From the trailhead parking, continue past the gate along the hiker-only road that switchbacks gradually up the east side of the ridge. At 0.3 mile, the trail intersects Elmore Mountain Trail; continue straight through this intersection, following signs for Fire Tower Trail.

Continue up Fire Tower Trail for 1.0 mile to a rocky ledge viewpoint to the east. This is a great spot to eat lunch as the fire tower itself has limited space picnicking. Families with toddlers may choose to turn back at this point.

The next 0.25 mile to the summit is the more challenging part of the loop. The route climbs over some steep, rocky sections, some with hand and foot-

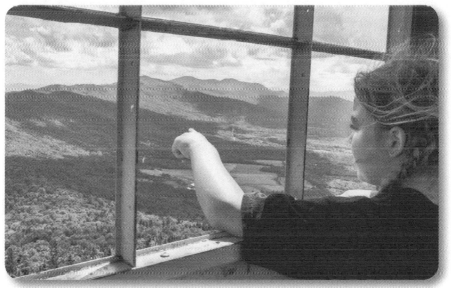

*The five-story fire tower that is perched on the summit
of Elmore Mountain offers exhilarating views!*

holds carved into the rock itself. Past these, the trail reaches a T intersection with Elmore Mountain Trail; continue straight to the fire tower on the left. From the top of the tower, look for the Worcester Range to the south and Mount Mansfield—the highest point in Vermont—to the west.

To descend, hike back down Fire Tower Trail to the T intersection with Elmore Mountain Trail. Veer left here to continue your clockwise loop. About 0.5 mile down the ridge, an interesting boulder field on the right begs to be explored. Our family spent a good part of an hour playing and hiding in its shady grottoes. Continue on down the trail to the aptly-named Balancing Rock, a great example of a glacial erratic (see Glacial Erratics).

The blue-blazed trail winds its way down the spine of the ridge, through soft hemlock forests and several mossy glens and wetlands. Eventually it reconnects with Fire Tower Trail at the intersection you passed on the way up. Turn left here and continue down the road to the trailhead.

PLAN B: The grassy campground at Elmore State Park makes a wonderful place to stay and explore for the weekend (or a week), with swimming, waterfalls, and hiking nearby. (Note: Dogs are not permitted on the park's beach.) The nearby Cabot Creamery in Cabot offers fine factory tours with unlimited free samples of delicious Vermont cheese at the end. Numerous waterfalls and swimming holes are within a 20-minute drive: Terrill Gorge in Morrisville and Jeff's Falls and Brewster Gorge, both in Johnson.

NEARBY: Nearby Morrisville is full of restaurants and stores mostly within a stone's throw of VT 100, including the Bee's Knees, which serves locally sourced foods from its own farm, along with live music and children's sing-a-longs. Check the schedule online at thebeesknees-vt.com.

GLACIAL ERRATICS

A glacial erratic is a large rock or boulder that has been transported to its current location by a glacier during an ice age that began two million years ago. They are easy to recognize because they often just don't fit in with their surroundings and are frequently spotted balancing in the forest or on top of a rocky ledge where they were left when the giant glaciers melted. Glacial erratics are usually much larger than the surrounding rocks and may even be a different type of rock entirely since they were moved from somewhere else.

Trip 73

All Ages $ 🐕   🛶   🏊   ⛺

Green River Reservoir

Paddle through remote and undeveloped Vermont wilderness to quiet and secluded backcountry campsites.

Address: Green River Dam Road, Hyde Park
Difficulty: Easy–Moderate
Distance: 1.0–7.0 miles, round-trip
Hours: No posted hours, Memorial Day weekend–Columbus Day weekend
Fee: $3 adults, $2 children ages 4–14
Contact: Green Mountain Reservoir State Park, 802-888-1349, 888-409-7579 (reservations January–May), vtstateparks.com/htm/grriver.htm
Bathrooms: None
Water/Snacks: None
Maps: USGS Morrisville and Eden quads; vtstateparks.com/pdfs/grriver.pdf
Directions by Car: From intersection of VT 108 and VT 100 in Stowe, head north on VT 100 for 8.9 miles to Morrisville and make a slight left onto VT 15A/Park Street. In 1.7 miles, turn right on VT 15 then make an immediate left onto Garfield Road. In 3.1 miles, follow Garfield Road as it makes a sharp right, then make an immediate left onto Green River Dam Road. Follow this for 1.3 miles to Green Mountain Reservoir State Park and the obvious boat launch (44° 37.269′ N, 72° 31.613′ W).

The Green River Reservoir (GRR) is like no other Vermont State Park. Unlike its well-developed and highly tended sister parks, the GRR is a wild, untamed place. The reservoir's undeveloped shoreline is a rarity in New England, and thanks to the acquisition of the land by the state in 1999, it is now protected as wildlife habitat and a recreation paradise.

These quiet waters hold immeasurable treasures for families: quiet misty-morning paddles, crackling campfires along the shoreline with fresh-caught fish for dinner, loons calling across the water on quiet starry nights.

The reservoir is officially designated as a "quiet lake," meaning no internal combustion engines, Jet Skis, or float planes are allowed. The effect is clear: no wakes, peaceful paddling, and the immense quiet that descends on a place with no machinery. Kayaks and canoes rule. Children will find it magical;

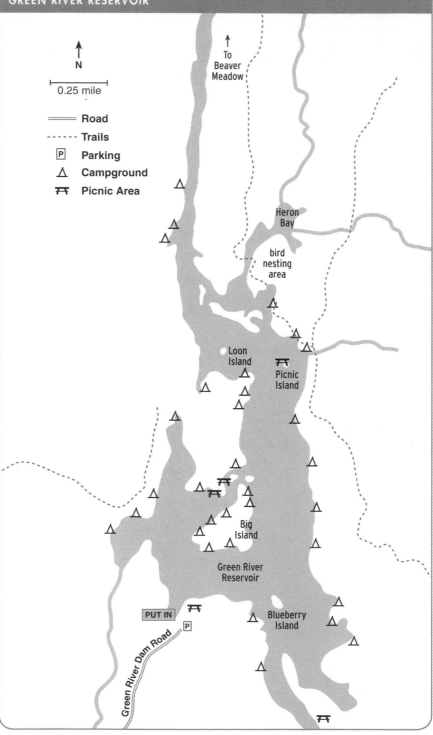

GREEN RIVER RESERVOIR

N

0.25 mile

Road
Trails
P Parking
△ Campground
🏕 Picnic Area

To
Beaver
Meadow

Heron
Bay

bird
nesting
area

Loon
Island

Picnic
Island

Big
Island

Green River
Reservoir

PUT IN
P

Blueberry
Island

Green River Dam Road

adults simply won't want to go home. The nearest canoe and kayak rentals are available at outfitters in Stowe and Jeffersonville.

Plan to day-trip and picnic on a small island, or to experience GRR in its fullest, camp at one of the 34 backcountry paddle-in campsites. Once you have set up your "base camp," explore hidden bays and secret islands by boat, swim, fish, and watch the wildlife that call this place home. We have seen many loons here, and moose love these secluded and quiet bodies of water. Make sure you explore the upper reaches of the Green River as it empties into the reservoir. As you paddle past campsite 13 at the north end, the banks get narrower and narrower, offering an excellent vantage point to spot wildlife onshore or turtles basking in the sun.

If you're adventurous, plan a multiday expedition, traveling from campsite to campsite.

PLAN B: The nearby Elmore Mountain (Trip 72) is an excellent day hike to a fire tower that has impressive views of this mountainous farm country.

NEARBY: Nearby Morrisville is full of restaurants and stores mostly centered on VT 100, including the Bee's Knees, which serves locally sourced foods from its own farm, along with live music and children's sing-a-longs. Check the schedule online at thebeesknees-vt.com. The nearest canoe and kayak rentals are available at outfitters in Stowe and Jeffersonville.

Trip 74

Ages 5+ | $ | 🐕 | 🚶

Wheeler Mountain

This could be the perfect hike: mostly moderate climbing with short steep sections, sweeping views from wide-open ledges, and the thrilling adventure of scrambling up rocky slabs.

Address: Wheeler Mountain Road (between US 5 and Big Valley Lane), Sutton
Difficulty: Moderate
Distance: 2.5 miles, round-trip
Hours: No posted hours
Fee: Free
Contact: Vermont Department of Forest, Parks, and Recreation, St. Johnsbury District, 802-751-0136, vtfpr.org/lands/willoughby.cfm
Bathrooms: None
Water/Snacks: None
Maps: USGS Sutton quad; vtfpr.org/lands/willoughby/fig11.pdf
Directions by Car: From I-91, Exit 26, head south on US 5 for 9.8 miles (past Crystal Lake on the left) to Wheeler Mountain Road. Turn left on Wheeler Mountain Road and continue past Wheeler Pond on your right. After 2.0 miles, park at the small pull-off and the trailhead on your left. If the lot is full, park on the dirt road itself, but be sure to pull completely off of the road (44° 43.677′ N, 72° 5.776′ W).

Similar to New Hampshire's Welch and Dickey mountains (Trip 33), Mount Wheeler offers quintessential slab hiking to gorgeous views over the surrounding landscape. The short distance combined with the exposed nature of the approach makes for an unforgettable experience for families. Much of Wheeler Mountain is on private land, but recreational use has been permitted by the landowners. Please continue to respect the private property and stay on the trail. Two trails approach the summit: Red Trail is steeper with open slabs, and White Trail is more gentle. We describe a counterclockwise loop ascending Red Trail and descending White Trail; if your younger hikers may struggle with steep grades, summit and descend via White Trail instead.

From the trailhead, follow the trail for a short distance through the woods and an overgrown yet beautiful meadow to the Red Trail intersection. Take a right onto Red Trail. Before long, a short, steep section traverses and climbs a

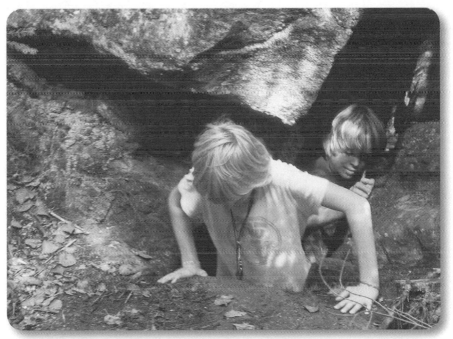

Even on hikes with the most amazing views or waterfalls, sometimes the highlight can be as simple as a cave or hiding spot you find along the way!

small cliff band; you may see rock climbers practicing on these beginner crags. Follow the base of the cliffs to the left as the trail steadily winds up a gradual section and crosses back over to the right. Keep your kids close; this section is exciting but steep. The views of Wheeler Pond are phenomenal as you gain elevation.

After you gain the top of the crag, the more gradual White Trail connects from the left. Continue up to the right into the woods following both red and white blazes as you go. We had a great time hiding in the many rock crevices and small caves along this section.

At 1.0 mile, the trail emerges onto some open ledges, and continues ascending up a narrow exposed ridge to the left. Be careful here, and keep small kids close. After gaining the top of this exposed ridge, the path dives back into low, mossy woods reminiscent of a scene from *The Hobbit*. Some of our favorite landscapes are these lush, mossy spruce forests that thrive on ridge tops throughout New England. Plan to lunch and siesta at Eagle Rock (1.25 miles), a fine block that juts off the north side of the mountain overlooking the fjord-like Lake Willoughby to the east.

As you descend, skip the cutoff for Red Trail on the left and simply continue back to the trailhead on White Trail. Along the way, the trail passes the ruins of an old maple sugaring operation in a mossy grove, where you can imagine what life may have been like here 100 years ago.

PLAN B: A lovely 1.6-mile trail winds around Wheeler Pond on Wheeler Mountain Road, and the Green Mountain Club maintains two year-round cabins on its shores. While the cabins don't offer electricity, they are heated and are a perfect rustic pond-side getaway in this beautiful and remote corner of Vermont. Call 802-244-7037 to make a reservation.

NEARBY: There are several eateries just south of Wheeler Mountain Road in West Burke and Lyndonville, both south on US 5.

Trip 75

Burnt Mountain

This remote, relatively unknown mountain leads you past beaver ponds, a high-mountain orchard, and a craggy summit.

Address: Rossier Road, Montgomery
Distance: 4.8 miles, round-trip
Difficulty: Moderate
Hours: No posted hours, May 15–December 15; welcome center open weekdays 9 A.M.–4 P.M., weekends 9 A.M.–5 P.M.; all trails closed April 15–May 15
Fee: Free for day use in summer and fall; contact Hazen's Notch Association for winter trail pass and rental fees
Contact: Hazen's Notch Association, 802-326-4799, hazensnotch.org/Hiking.htm
Bathrooms: None
Water/Snacks: None
Maps: USGS Hazen's Notch quad; hazensnotch.org/Winter-Trail-Map.htm
Directions by Car: From the intersection of VT 118 and VT 58, head east on VT 118 along the banks of the Trout River. After 2.1 miles, turn right on Rossier Road and follow this narrow lane for 0.5 mile to the parking area and trailhead kiosk at the old farm at the end of the road (44° 51.676′ N, 72° 34.644′ W).

Hazen's Notch is home to remote and beautiful hiking and world-class, groomed cross-country ski trails. Consider this trip for any season, though note that trail pass fees apply in winter; cross-country skis and snowshoes may be rented at the welcome center. At the trailhead, stop to check the kiosk on the right for trail updates and information about the Hazen's Notch Association, which manages this land. Started in 1994, the association is a prime example of a community-based land trust formed to preserve habitat and recreational activities.

From the trailhead, Beaver Ponds Trail starts as a wide woods road for the first mile and passes a series of beaver ponds on the right. Be prepared to get your feet wet: the very active beaver population creates ponds anywhere they can, often flooding the path, forcing hikers through ankle-deep water. (See Trip 10, About Beavers, for more information.)

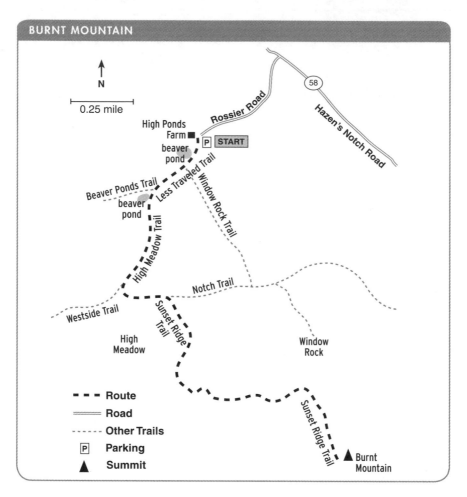

BURNT MOUNTAIN

N

0.25 mile

High Ponds Farm ■
P START
beaver pond
Rossier Road
58
Hazen's Notch Road
Less Traveled Trail
Window Rock Trail
Beaver Ponds Trail
beaver pond
High Meadow Trail
Notch Trail
Westside Trail
Sunset Ridge Trail
High Meadow
Window Rock
Sunset Ridge Trail
▲ Burnt Mountain

- - - Route
=== Road
----- Other Trails
P Parking
▲ Summit

Beaver Ponds Trail then enters High Meadow (0.5 mile), a historic apple orchard that is now maintained as a semi-wild meadow full of wildflowers, and
apple trees—and likely more than a few fairies, forest nymphs, and gnomes.
This is a great picnic and turnaround spot if the little ones are tired; from here,
the trail starts to climb up into the high country. Look for the summit of Burnt
Mountain looming above the meadow—the path heads all the way up there!

Follow High Meadow Trail through the meadow and stay left at the in-
tersection with Westside Trail, and right at the intersection with Notch Trail.
After another 0.25 mile on the Notch Trail the trail meets steeper and rockier
Sunset Ridge Trail.

The footpath climbs steadily up switchbacks through a maple and birch
forest. This section is short and steep; take plenty of quick breaks and have
some chocolate handy to keep motivation high. The reward at the top is worth
it! Finally, the trail tops out on Burnt Mountain Ridge, traverses its length and
the forested summit, and reaches the lookout rocks on the southern flank of

the mountain (2.4 miles). Look for Mount Mansfield (Trip 71) to the south. Return the way you came.

PLAN B: There is a serene and sandy swimming hole on the Trout River just below the Longley Bridge on VT 118 in between Montgomery Center and Montgomery.

NEARBY: Find great delis and restaurants in nearby Montgomery.

INFORMATION & RESOURCES

Recommended Maps

DeLorme's *Atlas and Gazetteer* series, available at outdoor outfitters and gas stations throughout New England, delorme.com

Connecticut River Paddlers' Trail, connecticutriverpaddlerstrail.org

Appalachian Mountain Club maps (Maine and New Hampshire), amcstore.outdoors.org/books-maps/maps

Green Mountain Club maps (Vermont), greenmountainclub.org

Recommended Books

White Mountain Guide by Steve Smith (AMC Books)

Quiet Water Maine by John Hayes and Alex Wilson (AMC Books)

Quiet Water New Hampshire and Vermont by John Hayes and Alex Wilson (AMC Books)

AMC Guide to Winter Hiking and Camping by Lucas St.Clair and Yemaya Mauer (AMC Books)

New England Waterfalls by Greg Parsons and Kate B. Watson (Countryman Press)

General

Appalachian Mountain Club, 603-466-2721, outdoors.org

Guide You Outdoors (basic outdoor skills), youtube.com/user/GuideYouOutdoors

Maine Resources

Acadia National Park, 207-288-3338, nps.gov/acad

Baxter State Park, 207-723-5140, baxterstateparkauthority.com

Maine Appalachian Trail Club, matc.org

Maine Audubon Society, 207-781-2330, maineaudubon.org

Maine Bureau of Parks and Lands, 207-287-3821, maine.gov/doc/parks

Maine Land Trust Network, 207-729-7366, mltn.org

Maine State Park Camping, 800-332-1501 or 207-624-9950, campwithme.com

Maine Tourism, 888-624-6345, visitmaine.com

Natural Resources Council of Maine, 800-287-2345, maineenvironment.org

The Nature Conservancy, 207-729-5181, nature.org/maine

Portland Trails, 207-775-2411, trails.org

New Hampshire Resources

Lakes Region Conservation Trust, 603-253-3301, lrct.org

New Hampshire Audubon, 603-224-9909, nhaudubon.org

New Hampshire State Parks, 603-271-3556, nhstateparks.org

Society for the Protection of New Hampshire Forests, 603-224-9945, forestsociety.org

Squam Lakes Association, 603-968-7336, squamlakes.org
White Mountain National Forest, 603-536-6100, fs.usda.gov/whitemountain

Vermont Resources
Cross Vermont Trail Association, 802-498-0079, crossvermont.org
Green Mountain Club, 802-244-7037, greenmountainclub.org
Green Mountain National Forest, 802-747-6700, fs.usda.gov/greenmountain
Local Motion, 802-652-2453, localmotion.org
Vermont State Parks, 888-409-7579, vtstateparks.com
Windmill Hill Pinnacle Association, 802-869-2071, windmillhillpinnacle.org

INDEX

ABOUT THE AUTHORS

Ethan Hipple's passion for the outdoors was ignited as a teenager working on a trail crew for the Student Conservation Association (SCA). He served as a croo member in the Appalachian Mountain Club's High Huts, guided trips for Prescott College, was an SCA Trail Crew Leader, and eventually ran the Western Region of the SCA High School Program. He has directed the New Hampshire Conservation Corps and is currently the Director of Parks and Recreation in Wolfeboro, New Hampshire. Along the way, he moonlit as a rickshaw driver, pizza bike-delivery driver, and street musician. He lives in Tuftonboro, New Hampshire, with his lovely wife, Sarah, and two awesome kids, where they love to find secret swimming holes, fish, kayak, surf, and play music on the porch. His favorite backcountry meal is Pozole Pie (Mexican-style lasagna cooked in a Dutch oven); the backcountry gear he cannot live without is a good umbrella.

Yemaya St.Clair grew up exploring the woods and waters of Puget Sound before discovering backpacking as a teenager and taking to the mountains. Her outdoor pursuits have taken her everywhere from the summits of Mount Rainier and Katahdin to the fjords of Patagonia and the canopy of Costa Rica. She worked as an environmental educator with the Student Conservation Association before turning her focus to freelance writing. This is her second guidebook for the AMC. She lives in Portland, Maine, with her husband, Lucas, and their two small kids, who came along on hiking, biking, and paddling trips before they could roll over.

APPALACHIAN MOUNTAIN CLUB

At AMC, connecting you to the freedom and exhilaration of the outdoors is our calling. We help people of all ages and abilities to explore and develop a deep appreciation of the natural world.

AMC helps you get outdoors on your own, with family and friends, and through activities close to home and beyond. With chapters from Maine to Washington, D.C., including groups in Boston, New York City, and Philadelphia, you can enjoy activities like hiking, paddling, cycling, and skiing, and learn new outdoor skills. We offer advice, guidebooks, maps, and unique lodges and huts to inspire your next outing. You will also have the opportunity to support conservation advocacy and research, youth programming, and caring for 1,800 miles of trails.

We invite you to join us in the outdoors.

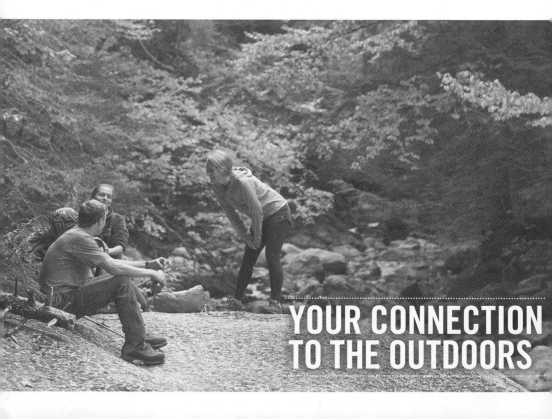

YOUR CONNECTION TO THE OUTDOORS

AMC IN NORTHERN NEW ENGLAND

AMC's northernmost chapters—Maine and New Hampshire—offer hundreds of outdoor activities year-round, including family-friendly trips and young member programs. Members maintain local trails, lead outdoor skills workshops, and promote stewardship of the region's natural resources. To view a list of AMC activities across the Northeast, visit activities.outdoors.org.

For decades, AMC has also been committed to conservation and sustainable forestry across the Northern Forest, which encompasses 26 million acres across Maine, New Hampshire, Vermont, and New York. AMC partners closely with the White Mountain National Forest on trail maintenance and alpine plant monitoring, and operates its huts and Pinkham Notch Visitor Center under a special use permit. Through its Maine Woods Initiative, AMC has permanently protected 66,500 acres of forestland while creating new opportunities for nature-based tourism through its Maine Wilderness Lodges. The Maine Woods Initiative seeks to address regional ecological and economic needs through outdoor recreation, resource protection, sustainable forestry, and community partnerships.

To learn more about AMC's regional conservation efforts, visit outdoors.org/conservation/wherewework.

AMC BOOK UPDATES

AMC Books strives to keep our guidebooks as up-to-date as possible to help you plan safe and enjoyable adventures. If after publishing a book we learn that trails have been relocated or route or contact information has changed, we will post the updated information online. Before you hit the trail, check for updates at outdoors.org/bookupdates.

While enjoying a trip from this book, if you notice discrepancies with the trip description or map, or if you find any other errors, please let us know by submitting them to amcbookupdates@outdoors.org or in writing to Books Editor, c/o AMC, 5 Joy Street, Boston, MA 02108. We will verify all submissions and post key updates each month. AMC Books is dedicated to being a recognized leader in outdoor publishing. Thank you for your participation.

NEW!

kids.outdoors.org

Hundreds of places to get outdoors close to home in Boston, New York City, Philadelphia, **and now in Maine, New Hampshire, and Vermont!**

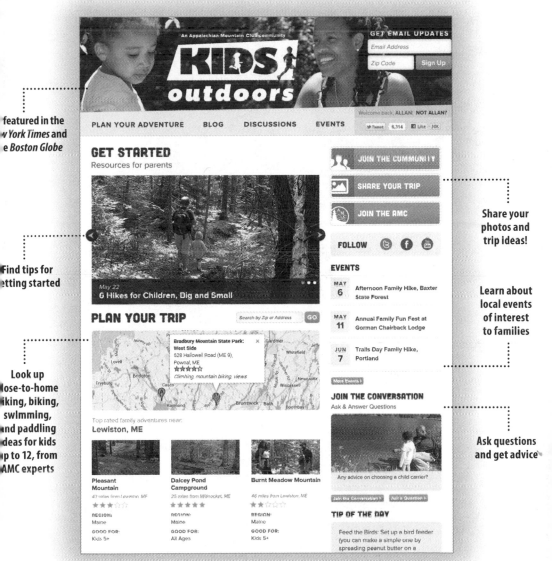

featured in the *New York Times* and *the Boston Globe*

Find tips for getting started

Look up close-to-home hiking, biking, swimming, and paddling ideas for kids up to 12, from AMC experts

Share your photos and trip ideas!

Learn about local events of interest to families

Ask questions and get advice

Join this FREE community today and share it with your friends.
Based on AMC's *Outdoors with Kids* guidebook series.

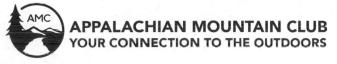

APPALACHIAN MOUNTAIN CLUB
YOUR CONNECTION TO THE OUTDOORS

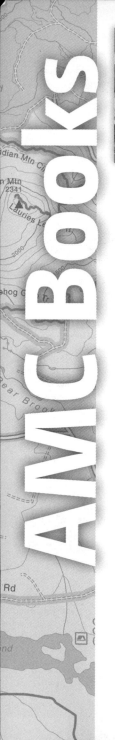
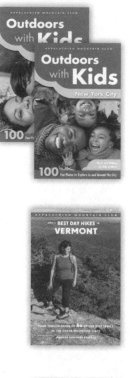
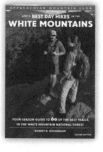
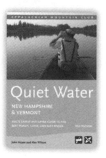

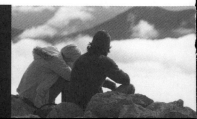